ACSM'S SPORTS MEDICINE REVIEW

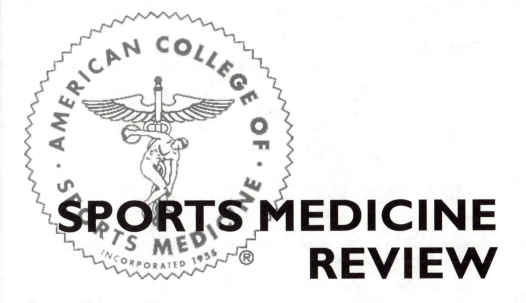

SPORTS MEDICINE REVIEW

Edited by

Robert E. Sallis, MD, FAAFP
Director of Research, Family Medicine Residency and Kaiser
    Permanente/SPORT Fellowship Programs
Kaiser Permanente Medical Center
Team Physician, Pomona College
Fontana, California

Murray E. Allen, MD
Consultant, Musculoskeletal-Sports Medicine
Chief Examiner in Sports Medicine,
    American Academy Sports Physicians
Chief Examiner in Sports Medicine,
    CAQ Board Review Course
American College of Sports Medicine
North Vancouver, British Columbia
CANADA

Ferdy Massimino, MD, MPH, FACSM
Clinical Practice Guideline Implementation and Clinical
    Education, Regional Occupational Health
Emergency Medicine/Sports Medicine
The Permanente Medical Group, Inc.
Oakland, California

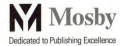
Mosby
Dedicated to Publishing Excellence

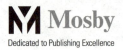

Mosby

Dedicated to Publishing Excellence

A Times Mirror Company

Vice President and Publisher: Anne S. Patterson
Editor: Robert Hurley
Developmental Editor: Lauranne Billus
Editorial Assistant: Marla Sussman
Project Manager: Linda Clarke
Production Editor: Jennifer Harper
Designer: Carolyn O'Brien
Manufacturing Supervisor: Andrew Christensen
Cover Photo: Philip and Karen Smith/Tony Stone Images
ACSM Group Publisher: D. Mark Robertson

Printed in the United States of America
Composition by Compset
Printing/binding by Malloy Lithographing, Inc.

Mosby–Year Book, Inc.
11830 Westline Industrial Drive
St. Louis, Missouri 63146

Library of Congress Cataloging-in-Publication Data

ACSM'S Sports Medicine Review / edited by Murray Allen.
    p. cm.
    Companion v. to: ACSM'S Essentials of Sports Medicine/edited by Robert
      Sallis, Ferdy Massimino, Murray Allen. c1997.
    ISBN 0-8151-0392-1 (alk. paper)
    1. Sports medicine—Examinations, questions, etc. I. Sallis, Robert;
Massimino, Ferdy; Allen, Murray.   II. Essentials of sports medicine.
    [DNLM: 1. Sports Medicine. 2. Athletic Injuries. QT 261 S767 1996]
  RC1210.E782 1996 Suppl.
  617.1'027'076—dc20
  DNLM/DLC
  for Library of Congress   96-6218
                                                                CIP

97 98 99 00 01 / 9 8 7 6 5 4 3 2 1

CONTRIBUTORS

Murray E. Allen, MD
Consultant, Musculoskeletal-Sports Medicine
Chief Examiner in Sports Medicine, American Academy Sports Physicians
Chief Examiner in Sports Medicine, CAQ Board Review Course
American College Sports Medicine
North Vancouver, British Columbia
CANADA

David V. Anderson, MD
Director, Orthopaedic Sports Medicine
Kaiser Permanente/SPORT Fellowship Program
Clinical Instructor, Loma Linda University
Fontana, California

Raul Artal, MD, FACSM
Professor and Chairman, Department of Obstetrics and Gynecology
SUNY Health Science Center
Syracuse and Crous Irving Memorial Hospital
Syracuse, New York

Evan S. Bass, MD
Department of Family Medicine and Sports Medicine
Kaiser Permanente
Gardena, California

Mark E. Batt, MB, BChir, MRCGP, Dip Sports Med
Senior Lecturer/Honorary Consultant in Sports Medicine
University of Nottingham
Centre for Sports Medicine
Department of Orthopaedic & Accident Surgery
University Hospital, Queen's Medical Centre
Nottingham, United Kingdom

David E.J. Bazzo, MD
Assistant Clinical Professor of Family Medicine
University of California, San Diego
Clinical Director, UCSD Medical Group
San Diego, California

Mark D. Bracker, MD
Associate Clinical Professor
University of California, San Diego
San Diego, California

Philip J. Buckenmeyer, MD
University Instructional Specialist
Research Director, Women's Wellness Center
SUNY Health Science Center/Dept of OB/GYN
Syracuse, New York

Walter L. Calmbach, MD
Assistant Professor
University of Texas Health Science Center
Director, Family Practice Sports Medicine Fellowship
Department of Family Practice
University Hospital
San Antonio, Texas

Robert C. Cantu, MA, MD, FACS, FACSM
Medical Director, National Center for Catastrophic Sports Injury Research
    Chapel Hill, North Carolina
Chief, Neurosurgery Service
Director, Service of Sports Medicine
Emerson Hospital
Concord, Massachusetts

C. Mark Chassay, MD
Graduate, Kaiser Permanente/SPORT Fellowship Program and Team
    Physician, The University of Texas Department of Intercollegiate
    Athletics for Women
Austin, Texas

Andrew J. Cole, MD, FACSM
Clinical Assistant Professor, Department of Physical Medicine and
    Rehabilitation
Clinical Assistant Professor, Department of Physical Therapy
University of Texas Southwestern Medical Center
Director, Spine Rehabilitation Services
Baylor University Medical Center
Department of Physical Medicine and Rehabilitation,
    Tom Landry Sports Medicine and Research Center
Dallas, Texas

Ellen J. Coleman, MA, MPH, RD
Nutrition Consultant
The Sport Clinic
Riverside, California

Mitchell W. Craib, PhD
Professor of Sports Studies
Guilford College
Greensboro, North Carolina

Robert J. Dimeff, MD
Medical Director, Section of Sports Medicine
Department of Orthopaedic Surgery
Cleveland Clinic Foundation
Clinical Professor, Family Practice
Case Western Reserve University
Cleveland, Ohio
Associate Professor, Department of Family Medicine
The Ohio State University
Columbus, Ohio

E. Randy Eichner, MD, FACSM
Professor of Medicine, University of Oklahoma Health Sciences Center
University Hospital and VAMC
Oklahoma City, Oklahoma

Wade F. Exum, MD, MBA
Preceptor, USOG/Glaxo Pharm. D. Fellowship
USOG Director of Drug Control Administration
Olympic Training Center
Colorado Springs, Colorado

Allen C. Felix, MD
Instructor, Kaiser Permanente/SPORT Fellowship Program
Family Physician, The SPORT Clinic
Riverside, California

Karl B. Fields, MD
Associate Professor, Dept of Family Medicine
Director Family Practice Resident
Moses Cone Health System
Greensboro, North Carolina

James G. Garrick, MD, FACSM
Director, Center for Sports Medicine
Saint Francis Memorial Hospital
San Francisco, California

Peter G. Gerbino II, MD
Assistant Professor of Orthopaedic Surgery
University of Cincinnati
Division of Sports Medicine
Cincinnati, Ohio

Thomas J. Gill, MD
Clinical Fellow, Harvard Medical School
Department of Orthopedic Surgery
Massachusetts General Hospital
Boston, Massachusetts

Jorge Gomez, MD
Assistant Professor
Department of Pediatrics
University of Texas Health Science Center
Team Physician, San Antonio Pumas
University Hospital
San Antonio, Texas

Gary A. Green, MD, FACSM
Clinical Assistant Professor
University of California, Los Angeles, Division of Family Medicine
Assistant Team Physician, UCLA Intercollegiate Athletics
UCLA Medical Center
Los Angeles, California

Sally S. Harris, MD, MPH
Stanford University Team Physician
Pediatrician and Sports Medicine Specialist
Palo Alto Medical Clinic
Palo Alto, California

Stanley A. Herring, MD, FACSM
Clinical Associate Professor, Department of Rehabilitation Medicine
Clinical Associate Professor, Department of Orthopaedics
University of Washington
Puget Sound Sports and Spine Physicians
Seattle, Washington

Greg Hoeksema, MD
Clinical Staff, University of California, San Diego
Head, Marine Corps Recruit Depot Medical Clinic
Director, Sports Medicine Clinic
Naval Medical Center
San Diego, California

David O. Hough, MD, FACSM
Professor, Family Practice
Director, Sports Medicine
Head Team Physician, Michigan State University
East Lansing, Michigan

Jeffrey A. Housner, MD
Clinical Instructor and Sports Medicine Fellow
University of California, Los Angeles, Division of Family Medicine
UCLA Center for Health Sciences
Los Angeles, California

Michael D. Jackson, MD
Midwest Rehabilitation Physicians
Golden Valley, Michigan

Mimi D. Johnson, MD, FACSM
Clinical Assistant Professor, Division of Adolescent Medicine
Department of Pediatrics
Assistant Team Physician, University of Washington
Seattle, Washington
Washington Sports Medicine
Kirkland, Washington

Robert J. Johnson, MD, FACSM
Director, Primary Care Sports Medicine
Department of Family Practice, Hennepin County Medical Center
Family Medical Center
Minneapolis, Minnesota

Kirk Jones, MS, ATC
Associate Professor, Physical Education
Pomona College
NATA, ACSM
Claremont, California

Todd Jorgenson, MD
Graduate, Kaiser Permanente/SPORT Fellowship Program
Kaiser Permanente Medical Center
Fontana, California

W. Benjamin Kibler, MD, FACSM
Medical Director
Lexington Clinic Sports Medicine Center
Lexington, Kentucky

William D. Knopp, MD
Director of Sports Medicine, MacNeal F.P. Residency Program
MacNeal Hospital/Rush Medical School
Clinical Faculty, MacNeal Hospital
Berwyn, Illinois

Robert L. Kronisch, MD
Staff Physician
Sports Medicine Consultant, Student Health Service
San Jose State University
San Jose, California

Ferdy Massimino, MD, MPH, FACSM
Clinical Practice Guideline Implementation and Clinical Education,
    Regional Occupational Health
    Emergency Medicine/Sports Medicine
The Permanente Medical Group, Inc.
Oakland, California

Angus M. McBryde, Jr., MD
Professor and Chairman
The Medical University of South Carolina
Department of Orthopaedic Surgery
Division of Sports Medicine
Charleston, South Carolina

Roger L. McCoy, II, MD
Team Physician
Arizona State University
Family Practice/Sports Medicine
Arizona Orthopedics and Sports Medicine Specialists Sportsclub
Phoenix, Arizona

Douglas B. McKeag, MD, MS, FACSM
Formerly: Professor of Family Practice
Coordinator of Sports Medicine, Michigan State University Family Practice
East Lansing, Michigan
Currently: Professor and Vice Chairman Family Medicine and
Orthopaedic Surgery
Director of Primary Care Sports Medicine
Musculoskeletal Institute
University of Pittsburgh Medical Center
Pittsburgh, Pennsylvania

Lyle J. Micheli, MD, FACSM
Associate Clinical Professor of Orthopaedic Surgery
Harvard Medical School
Director, Division of Sports Medicine
Children's Hospital
Boston, Massachusetts

James L. Moeller, MD
Assistant Professor of Orthopaedic Surgery
Primary Care Sports Medicine
Department of Orthopaedics
University of Pittsburgh
Pittsburgh, Pennsylvania

James M. Moriarity, MD
Physician, University Health Services
University of Notre Dame
Notre Dame, Indiana

Aurelia Nattiv, MD
Assistant Clinical Professor
UCLA, Division of Family Medicine
Department of Orthopaedic Surgery
Assistant Team Physician, UCLA
Los Angeles, California

Steven R. Neish, MD, FACSM
Assistant Professor of Pediatrics
University of Colorado
Pediatric Cardiologist
Fitzsimons Army Medical Center
Aurora, Colorado

Andrew W. Nichols, MD, FACSM
Associate Professor, Department of Family Practice and Community Health
John A. Burns School of Medicine, University of Hawaii at Manoa
Team Physician
University of Hawaii at Manoa
Honolulu, Hawaii

Carol L. Otis, MD, FACSM
Adjunct Assistant Professor, Internal Medicine
Director, Specialty Clinics
University of California, Los Angeles, Student Health Services
Los Angeles, California

William Parham, PhD, ABPP
Associate Director, Clinical and COPE Services
UCLA, Student Psychological Services
Los Angeles, California

Herbert G. Parris, MD
Assistant Clinical Professor
University of Colorado School of Medicine
Teaching Faculty
St. Joseph Hospital Family Practice Residency Program
St. Joseph Hospital
The Denver Center for Sports/Family Medicine
Denver, Colorado

Peter B. Raven, PhD, FACSM
Professor and Chair
Department of Physiology
University of North Texas Health Science Center
Fort Worth, Texas

Troy Reese, PharmD
Resident Pharmacist
United States Olympic Committee
Colorado Springs, Colorado

E. Lee Rice, DO, FACSM
Clinical Professor of Family Practice & Sports Medicine
College of Osteopathic of the Pacific
Pomona, California
Assistant Clinical Professor, University of California San Diego School of Medicine
Department of Community and Family Medicine
San Diego Sports Medicine, Orthopaedics and Family Health Center
San Diego, California

Brent S.E. Rich, MD, ATC
Team Physician, Arizona State University
Private Practice, Arizona Orthopaedic and Sports Medicine Specialists
Phoenix, Arizona

David B. Richards, MD
Orthopedic Surgeon and Sports Medicine Physician
Lexington Clinic Sports Medicine Center
Lexington, Kentucky

Michael E. Robinson, MD
Primary Care Sports Medicine, Department of Orthopedics
The Permanente Medical Group
Team Physician, United States Water Polo
Sacramento, California

Aaron L. Rubin, MD, FACSM
Director, Kaiser Permanente/SPORT Fellowship Program
Team Physician, Rubidoux High School
University of California, Riverside
Partner and Staff Physician, Department of Family Medicine
Kaiser Permanente Medical Center
Fontana, California

Anthony J. Saglimbeni, MD
Fellow, Primary Care Sports Medicine
Family and Preventive Medicine
University of California, San Diego
Clinical Instructor
University of California, San Diego Medical Center
San Diego, California

Robert E. Sallis, MD, FAAFP
Director of Research, Family Medicine Residency and Kaiser
  Permanente/SPORT Fellowship Programs
Kaiser Permanente Medical Center
Team Physician, Pomona College
Fontana, California

Warren Scott, MD
Clinical Instructor of Surgery
Stanford University Medical Center
Chief, Sports Medicine
Departments of Orthopedics and Emergency Medicine
Kaiser Permanente Medical Center
Santa Clara, California

Lauren M. Simon, MD, MPH
Assistant Professor of Family Medicine
Loma Linda University School of Medicine
Director, Sports Medicine Program
Loma Linda University Family Practice Residency Program
Loma Linda, California

Stephen M. Simons, MD, FACSM
Associate Clinical Professor, Family Medicine
Indiana University
Associate Director, Family Practice Residency
Saint Joseph's Medical Center
South Bend, Indiana

Angela D. Smith, MD, FACSM
Assistant Professor of Orthopaedics
Case Western Reserve University School of Medicine
University Hospitals
Cleveland, Ohio

Edward D. Snell, MD
Assistant Professor
Medical College of Pennsylvania and Hahnemann University
Primary Care Sports Medicine
Allegheny Orthopaedic Associates/Allegheny General-Duquesne
University Sports Medicine Institute
Allegheny General Hospital
Pittsburgh, Pennsylvania

Steven D. Stahle, MD
Associate Professor
St. Louis University School of Medicine
Director of Sports Medicine
Deaconess Health System
Family Medicine, Dept. Deaconess Hospital
St. Louis, Missouri

Jeffrey L. Tanji, MD
Associate Professor and Associate Director, Residency Program
Director, Sports Medicine Program
University of California, Davis, Medical Center
Sacramento, California

Suzanne M. Tanner, MD, FACSM
Assistant Professor, Department of Orthopedics and Pediatrics
University of Colorado Health Sciences Center
Director, Adolescent Sports Medicine
The Denver Children's Hospital
Denver, Colorado

Steven P. Van Camp, MD, FACSM
Professor, College of Professional Studies
San Diego State University
Assistant Clinical Professor, Department of Pathology
University of California, San Diego, School of Medicine
Alvarado Medical Group
San Diego, California

Craig Wargon, DPM
Diplomate American Board of Podiatric Surgery
Residency Director, Kaiser, Santa Clara
Kaiser Permanente
Santa Clara, California

J. Michael Wieting, DO, Med
Instructor, Department of Physical Medicine and Rehabilitation
Michigan State University — College of Osteopathic Medicine
Staff Physiatrist
Michigan State University Sports Medicine Center
Michigan Capital Medical Center
East Lansing, Michigan

Carl Winfield, MD
Staff Physician, Division of Sports Medicine
Naval Hospital
Camp Le Jeune, North Carolina

Robert A. Wiswell, MD
Associate Professor, Department of Exercise Sciences
University of Southern California
Los Angeles, California

PREFACE

The cornerstone for the delivery of quality health care today is the primary care physician. This reality is especially true in sports medicine, which encompasses a wide variety of disciplines. Although no single practitioner can provide all the care needed by an athlete, athletes do require a broadly trained physician as their point of first contact with the health care system. This physician should be able to care for most of the sports-related problems they encounter and effectively arrange and manage consultative care when needed.

This role is nothing new for the primary care physician. Virtually all primary care physicians practicing today are confronted with the sick or injured athlete on a regular basis. A major portion of the field of sports medicine is really nothing more than the primary care of athletes. That is not to say that athletes do not at times require specialized expertise. A primary care physician with additional training in sports medicine can fill a vital role in caring for athletes, whether as a team physician or by seeing patients in a sports medicine clinic.

The American Board of Medical Specialties has defined the field of sports medicine as a broad area of health care that includes:

1. Exercise as an essential component of health care throughout life;
2. Medical management and supervision of recreational and competitive athletes and all others who exercise; and
3. Exercise for prevention and treatment of disease and injury.

Based on this broad definition, a sports medicine physician should have a wide scope of training. For this reason, the major primary care specialties (family medicine, internal medicine, pediatrics, and emergency medicine) developed an examination to recognize competence in sports medicine. Passing this examination, which was first given in 1993, confers a Certificate of Added Qualifications (CAQ) in sports medicine. To sit for this examination, physicians must hold board certification in one of these primary care specialties, and must have completed a one year fellowship in sports medicine. A practice eligibility pathway is available through the 1999 examination.

The origins of these books, ACSM'S *Essentials of Sports Medicine* and ACSM'S *Sports Medicine Review,* began with a board review course for the first CAQ examination in sports medicine. This course was conceived and organized by our co-editor, Dr. Ferdy Massimino, and sponsored by the

American College of Sports Medicine (ACSM). It ranks as one of the College's most ambitious and broad based education efforts. This conference brought together a vast array of sports medicine experts from across the nation to cover the entire range of primary care sports medicine topics, and lasted 5½ days while encompassing over 50 hours of lecture time. The entire course was filmed by CME Video and released as a 27-tape, comprehensive review of sports medicine. A similar course was staged in conjunction with the American Academy of Family Physicians (AAFP) before the 1995 CAQ examination.

ACSM'S *Essentials of Sports Medicine* has sprung from the massive syllabus that accompanied these conferences. Most of the topics and many of the speakers from these conferences are represented here. Most authors are primary care physicians who are leaders in the practice and teaching of sports medicine across the country. Numerous specialists, well known for their care of athletes, have contributed to this book as well. All have a strong background in understanding the needs of and providing relevant information for primary care sports medicine physicians.

ACSM'S *Essentials of Sports Medicine* is divided into 3 sections and consists of 82 chapters. The first 31 chapters cover medical topics relevant to the athlete. The next 42 chapters deal with musculoskeletal topics as they relate to the athlete. The final 9 chapters cover sports-specific topics and include an integrated discussion of important medical and musculoskeletal problems unique to athletes who compete in these sports. All chapters are done in outline format to facilitate easy study as well as to provide a rapid reference source.

Although this book was initially conceived as review material for the CAQ examination in sports medicine, its appeal will be much broader than that. It should be of great benefit to any physician who wants a comprehensive review of or easy reference to sports medicine. It should also be useful to residents (whether in primary care, orthopedics, or physiatry) who need a focused study guide to accompany rotations in sports medicine.

The companion text to this book is titled ACSM'S *Sports Medicine Review.* Like *Essentials,* it originated from both the ACSM and AAFP review courses. Both of these courses included a daily mock board exam over the topics covered by the previous day's speakers. These examinations were graded each day and course participants were able to compare their scores with those of others taking the course.

Many of these questions, as well as numerous new ones, have been incorporated into the companion review text. With each question is a paragraph long answer explaining each of the choices. These questions correspond to the chapters in *Essentials* and highlight the important points of each chapter. These books should be used in combination and together provide an outstanding means of education and self assessment.

The education of primary care physicians is of vital importance to the American College of Sports Medicine. I believe the primary care physician is "where the rubber meets the road" in sports medicine. After the vast cadre of ACSM researchers and specialists advance sports medicine, the primary care physician takes this information and puts it into practice. Without well trained and receptive primary caregivers, the full benefit of the advances in sports medicine the College cultivates would not be realized. Our goal has been to help bridge this gap between new advances in sports medicine and their implementation.

I hope you will find these books useful in your sports medicine endeavors.

Robert Sallis, MD
Rancho Cucamonga, CA
1996

ACKNOWLEDGMENTS

On behalf of Dr. Allen, Dr. Massimino, and myself, I would like to thank all of the physicians and scientists who contributed the questions and answers which make up this book. Their dedication to the goals of the American College of Sports Medicine are evidenced by their work here. Thanks also to Mark Robertson at ACSM for all of his support. Bob Hurley and his staff at Mosby, including Lauranne Billus, Mia Carino, Marla Sussman, and Jennifer Harper have been wonderful to work with. Their hard work and professionalism has been greatly appreciated.

Special recognition goes to Murray Allen, MD for all of his hard work on this project. Murray has years of experience in composing sports medicine examinations, and this was invaluable in helping to ensure that the questions presented here are both relevant and educational.

Robert Sallis, MD

INTRODUCTION

"Ignorance ain't what you don't know, it's what you do know that ain't right"
Will Rogers
"How do I know what I should know, and how do I know that I know it?"
Murray Allen, 1996

Sports medicine has gone through a procession of identities, starting with the odd collection of hail-and-hardy athletic minded doctors, up to the current status of major international sports medicine organizations that are tied to many centers of higher learning. All have one thing in mind, the pursuit of excellence in the management of sports selective-specific disorders. The key to this pursuit is knowledge. But what knowledge? What are we supposed to know in order to function as a sports medicine doctor?

The pursuit of excellence is spread over a wide base. Most of us have attended the popular conferences, some of which have provided huge volumes of printed materials, enough to tax our weight limit on the flight home. With courage, when we open the binders, we find that sports medicine is a discipline that entails elements from almost all the specialties. Yet none of the specialties in themselves can cope with the health concerns of the athlete. In the companion book of this series, ACSM'S *Essentials of Sports Medicine*, Robert Sallis prefaced above that sports medicine was the realm of the primary care physician. Certainly if you agreed with Bob that general or primary practice required the broad based wisdom of Solomon, then you've pegged sports medicine.

There are some philosophical differences between general and sports medicine, but mostly in degree. The general or family doctor is often trying to pick the patient up off the floor, out of the depths of some illness. By contrast, the sports medicine doctor tries to pull the athlete off the ceiling, trying to nudge them off the wall of overuse. Both perspectives are trying to optimize their patient's function, which for the competitive athlete is crowding the fine line. But the general public would like to emulate their sports heroes, and if sports medicine is good for the athlete then it must be good for their fans. How often have we heard our non-athletic patient say, "you can fix the athlete, so please fix me!"

The latest trend in sports medicine was inevitable—the *"Certificate of Added Qualification"* (*CAQ*) in Sports Medicine. Examinations were bound to be the next frontier, as has been the case in all other disciplines. The first examinations in sports medicine were held by the American Academy of Sports Physicians (AASP) in 1985, a small group that held in-house tests of member skills. Since, other American and Canadian sports medicine organizations have developed various levels of sports medicine exams for their members, and offered various levels of qualification. None proffer "specialty" qualifications.

Examinations offer you a chance to test your skills, like the athlete lined up at the start, waiting for the gun. The athlete is timed over the distance, the CAQ tests your knowledge. Some win, some lose. In the sports field, when you're ready to compete, there are usually many trial runs, mock or lesser competitions that prepare you to compete in your chosen field. How do we make ourselves ready in sports medicine, ready for a test?

Few, or perhaps none, of us as medical practitioners can personally accumulate all the knowledge required through direct high volume contact with sports specific disorders. The day and age of the experienced renaissance man is over, there is simply too much to learn for any one person to learn it through exposure alone. However, through our vicarious exposure to the accumulated knowledge of others, we can truly function as near-experts on many topics. Conferences, workshops, texts, proceedings, audio and video tapes, and simulated examinations can help us arrive to the point where we can qualify as the sports medicine doctor. This last step is the CAQ exam. If you pass, all it provides is a simple piece of paper, but it infers a trusted base in sports medicine.

The following ACSM'S *Sports Medicine Review* is intended to act like a trial run. The self-examination method is a critical part of the preparation process. You might think you know it, but do you? No two people learn in the same manner, and written examinations are not true reality checks, but at least they provide data on some minimal knowledge set that presumes to represent reality. It is not sufficient as an ultimate test of knowledge, sometimes the brightest and wisest fail! Part of the problem is what is known as "examination skill." Some persons learn how to take exams, or somehow have the right knack. Do You? By testing yourself with this *Review,* you should spot your strong and weak points, and then re-focus where your studies will do the most good. You should also learn how to take an exam. It has been suggested that the student who knows how to take an exam has a 30% advantage over the equally knowledgeable student who is not exam-skilled. Familiarity with the exam process does not breed contempt, but it does breed confidence.

Each chapter in this *Review* is a set of questions related to the topic heading. Each chapter is mirrored by the same topic with the same companion chapter heading in the ACSM'S *Essentials of Sports Medicine*. Each author of the *Essentials* has picked the best questions that relate to the basic knowledge of the chapter, which now appear in the *Review*.

The *Review* offers you a chance to test your skills. Give it your best shot. A good study plan is to read an *Essentials* chapter, then take the exam questions in the same chapter in the *Review*. Correct your own exam, and if you did well, then move on to the next chapter. If you did poorly, then you need to do more work on that chapter; but *now you know what it is that you need to know.*

Saying thanks to all the persons who have helped to put this *Review* together would take up a whole chapter. However, the short list includes Bob Sallis and Ferdy Massimino who spearheaded the ACSM'S *Essentials of Sports Medicine*. The American College of Sports Medicine deserves special praise for supporting this project, and there were a lot of unsung heroes shepherding this project through the system. And Mosby has worked real hard in keeping the pace up, and softly encouraging us to make the deadlines. The editorial staff are the true heroes of any book, they did a lot of the grunt work, and this is no exception for the *Review*.

My own thanks go to my many students over the years, who took my examinations, and with their sometimes grumbling feedback, the good, the bad, and the ugly, finally taught me how to formulate the fair question. I hope some of those hard fought skills showed through in the examination questions you took in this *Review*.

But of course nothing happens without the accumulated wisdom of each chapter's author, that special expert in a focused area of sports medicine, that when combined with all the other experts, makes a book. This *Review* is a testimony to their hard work and dedication, we appreciate all that they could offer.

And finally to our wives, husbands, families, and friends, who at times may have wondered why we kept working so hard and so long into the night. Well, the final edition is our reward so I hope you enjoy the *Review*, eh!

Murray E. Allen, MD
North Vancouver, British Columbia
Canada
1996

CONTENTS

M E D I C A L   T O P I C S

Cardiology

1. Cardiac Rehabilitation, **2**
   Mark D. Bracker

2. Hypertension, **5**
   Jeffrey L. Tanji, Mark E. Batt, Murray E. Allen

3. Exercise Testing and Prescription, **9**
   Brent S. E. Rich

4. Cardiac Arrhythmias in the Athlete, **12**
   Steven R. Neish, Steven P. Van Camp

5. Sudden Death in Athletes, **15**
   Steven P. Van Camp

Hematology

6. Anemia and Blood Doping, **18**
   E. Randy Eichner

Infectious Disease

7. Human Immunodeficiency Virus, **21**
   E. Lee Rice, Murray E. Allen

8. Sexually Transmitted Disease, **26**
   James L. Moeller, David O. Hough

9. Infectious Disease in Athletes, **29**
   Herbert G. Parris

Pulmonary

10. Exercise-Induced Asthma, **32**
    Robert J. Johnson, Murray E. Allen

General Medicine

11. Care of the Diabetic Athlete, **35**
    James M. Moriarity

12. Gastrointestinal Problems in Athletes, **38**
    Jeffrey A. Housner, Gary A. Green

13. Genitourinary Problems, **42**
    Aaron L. Rubin

14. The Geriatric Athlete, **45**
    Edward D. Snell, Robert J. Dimeff

15. Dermatology, **48**
    William D. Knopp

16. Ear, Nose, and Throat Problems, **51**
    Allen C. Felix

17. Environmental Concerns
    17a. Heat, **54**
    Brent S. E. Rich

    17b. Hypothermia and Frostbite, **58**
    Murray E. Allen

    17c. Altitude Illness, **66**
    Ferdy Massimino

18. The Preparticipation Examination, **69**
    Robert E. Sallis

19. Exercise Physiology, **72**
    Peter B. Raven

20. Sports Psychology, **76**
    Aurelia Nattiv, William Parham

21. Nutrition in Sports, **79**
    Ellen J. Coleman

The Female Athlete

22. Exercise and Menstrual Function, **82**
    Carol L. Otis

23. Pregnancy, **85**
    Raul Artal, Philip J. Buckenmeyer, Robert A. Wiswell

24. The Female Athlete Triad, **90**
    Carol L. Otis

25. Osteoporosis, **95**
    Murray E. Allen

26. Eating Disorders, **98**
    Mimi D. Johnson

The Pediatric Athlete

27. Growth and Development Concerns for Prepubescent and Adolescent Athletes, **101**
    Suzanne M. Tanner

Drugs and Sports

28. Nonsteroidal Antiinflamma- tory Drugs, **104**
    Jeffrey L. Tanji, Mark E. Batt

29. Banned Substances and Drugs, **107**
    Wade F. Exum

30. Anabolic-Androgenic Steroids, **112**
    Wade F. Exum, Troy Reese

31. Illicit Drug Use in Sports, **116**
    William D. Knopp

MUSCULOSKELETAL TOPICS
Shoulder

32. Anatomy and Biomechanics of the Shoul- der, **120**
    Todd Jorgenson

33. History and Physical Examination of the Shoulder, **123**
    Greg Hoeksema

34. Impingement Syndrome and Rotator Cuff Injuries, **127**
    Anthony J. Saglimbeni, David E.J. Bazzo

35. Shoulder Instability, **132**
    Thomas J. Gill, Lyle J. Micheli

36. Brachial Plexus Injuries, **135**
    Robert E. Sallis

37. Rehabilitation of Shoulder Injuries, **138**
    David B. Richards, W. Benjamin Kibler

Elbow and Forearm

38. Anatomy and Biomechanics of the Elbow and Forearm, **141**
    Michael D. Jackson, Douglas B. McKeag

39. History and Physical Examination of the Elbow and Forearm, **144**
    Michael D. Jackson, Douglas B. McKeag

40. Injuries About the Elbow, **147**
    Walter L. Calmbach, Jorge Gomez

Wrist and Hand

41. History and Physical Exam, **150**
    Murray E. Allen

42. Wrist and Hand Injuries in Sports, **153**
    Robert J. Dimeff

Head Injuries

43. Diagnosis and Management of Concussion, **164**
    Robert C. Cantu

44. Field Management of Head Injuries and Return to Play, **167**
    Roger L. McCoy II

Cervical Spine Injuries

45. Anatomy and Biomechanics, **170**
    Evan S. Bass

46. Fractures and Dislocation of the Cervical Spine, **174**
    Evan S. Bass

47.   Extra axial Cervical Spine
       Injury, 177
       James M. Moriarity

48.   Cervical Spine Injuries: On-
       Field Management, 180
       Andrew W. Nichols

Lumbar Spine Injuries

49.   Low Back Pain, 184
       Robert J. Johnson, Murray E. Allen

50.   Spondylolysis and
       Spondylolisthesis, 187
       Lyle J. Micheli, Peter G. Gerbino, II

51.   Lumbar Spine Pain: Rehabili-
       tation and Return
       to Play, 192
       Andrew J. Cole, Stanley A. Herring

Knee and Hip

52.   Knee Anatomy and Mecha-
       nisms of Injury, 195
       David V. Anderson

53.   Knee Ligament Injuries, 198
       James G. Garrick

54.   Meniscal Injuries, 202
       James G. Garrick

55.   Anterior Knee Pain and
       Overuse, 205
       J. Michael Wieting, Douglas B. McKeag

56.   Rehabilitation of the Injured
       Knee, 210
       David B. Richards, W. Benjamin Kibler

57.   Anatomy and Examination of
       the Hip, 212
       Carl Winfield

58.   Common Hip Injuries, 215
       Carl Winfield

Ankle and Foot

59.   Ankle and Foot
       Anatomy, 218
       Aaron L. Rubin

60.   Ankle Ligament Injuries, 221
       Aaron L. Rubin

61.   Ankle Fractures in
       Athletes, 226
       Angus M. McBryde, Jr.

62.   Rehabilitation of Ankle
       Injuries, 229
       Stephen M. Simons

63.   Sports Injuries to the Feet,
       232
       Craig Wargon

64.   Biomechanics of Running and
       Gait, 235
       Karl B. Fields, Mitchell W. Craib

65.   Ankle Taping and
       Bracing, 243
       Kirk Jones

Pediatric Concerns

66.   Musculoskeletal Injuries
       Unique to Growing Children
       and Adolescents, 246
       Angela D. Smith

67.   Rehabilitation for Children
       and Adolescents, 252
       Angela D. Smith

68.   Strength Training for Children
       and Adolescents, 255
       Sally S. Harris

General Musculoskeletal Topics

69.   Fracture Diagnosis and
       Management of Common
       Injuries, 258
       Michael E. Robinson

70.   Overuse Injuries, 261
       Warren Scott

71.   Physiology of Musculoskeletal
       Growth, 264
       Mimi D. Johnson

72.   Finding and Correcting Flexi-
       bility Deficits for Injury
       Prevention and Rehabili-
       tation, 267
       Angela D. Smith

73.   Epidemiology of In-
       juries, 271
       James G. Garrick

Sports Specific Problems

74.   Injuries in Football and
       Soccer, 274
       James M. Moriarity

75.   Track and Field, 277
       Carol L. Otis, Murray E. Allen

76. Basketball Injuries, **280**
Michael D. Jackson, James L. Moeller,
David O. Hough

77. Bicycling Injuries, **283**
Robert L. Kronisch

78. Running, **287**
Karl B. Fields

79. Aquatic Sports, **290**
Lauren M. Simon

80. Overhand Throwing
Sports, **294**
Robert E. Sallis

81. Skiing Injuries, **297**
Steven D. Stahle, Robert J. Dimeff

82. Dance, **300**
C. Mark Chassay

MEDICAL TOPICS

CHAPTER **1**

Cardiac Rehabilitation

Mark D. Bracker, MD

QUESTIONS

1-1. Leisure time exercise patterns and health status among college alumni have shown how past and present exercise relate to coronary heart disease risk. Which of the following statements is *incorrect:*

  a. Alumni who reported vigorous sports activity had about a 27% less risk of CHD than those who did not.

  b. Alumni who reported engaging in light sports activity only had the same risk of CHD as those who played no sports at all.

  c. Athletes who gave up their former energetic routines tended to have a lower risk of CHD than did alumni who had never been active as student athletes.

  d. A physically active adulthood is associated with lower CHD rates.

1-2. All of the following statements are true EXCEPT:

  a. Five risk factors (adequate exercise, no cigarette smoking, weight control, no hypertension, no parental CHD) contribute independently to lowering the risk of CHD.

  b. Hypertension is the least potent clinical risk factor and is the least prevalent.

  c. Sedentary life-style is highly prevalent and percentagewise represents the greatest contribution to risk of CHD.

  d. There is a graded inverse relationship between total physical activity and mortality.

1-3. Which of the following is not an absolute contraindication for entry into cardiac rehabilitation:
  a. Unstable angina.
  b. Moderate or severe aortic stenosis.
  c. Use of a cardiac pacemaker.
  d. Resting ST segment displacement greater than 3 mm.

1-4. All the statements concerning cardiac monitoring during cardiac rehabilitation are true, EXCEPT:
  a. The use of continuous or intermittent monitoring for a specific patient is of little importance.
  b. High-risk patients require the most extensive ECG monitoring and clinical supervision.
  c. All cardiac programs should include monitoring of blood pressure, heart rate symptoms, and effort intolerance.

1-5. Which one of the following statements is correct:
  a. The benefit of exercise is due to improvement in cardiorespiratory fitness.
  b. All patients demonstrate significant improvement in cardiac risk factor reduction after completing a cardiac rehabilitation program.
  c. Strenuous physical activity may increase the HDL cholesterol fraction.
  d. Most patients in a cardiac rehabilitation program show improvement in body weight and skin fold thickness.

ANSWERS

1-1. c. Athletes who gave up their former energetic routines tended to have a lower risk of CHD than did alumni who had never been active as student athletes.

1-2. b. Hypertension is the least potent clinical risk factor and is the least prevalent.

1-3. c. Use of a cardiac pacemaker.

1-4. a. The use of continuous or intermittent monitoring for a specific patient is of little importance.

1-5. c. Strenuous physical activity may increase the HDC cholesterol fraction.

CHAPTER 2

Hypertension

Jeffrey L. Tanji, MD

Mark E. Batt, MB, BChir

Murray E. Allen, MD

QUESTIONS

2-1. Hypertension is a proven risk factor for which of the following diseases:
  a. Transient quadraparesis.
  b. Systemic lupus erythematosus (SLE).
  c. Myocardial infarction.
  d. Migraine headaches.
  e. Peptic ulcer disease.

2-2. All of the following mechanisms explain why exercise may benefit patients with high blood pressure, EXCEPT:
  a. Peripheral vasodilatory effect of exercise.
  b. Increased renin production.
  c. Relaxation response.
  d. Decrease in serum catecholamines.
  e. Decreased insulin resistance.

2-3. The following antihypertensive medication is relatively contraindicated in the exercising hypertensive individual:
  a. Nonselective beta-blockers.
  b. Angiotensin-converting enzyme (ACE) inhibitors.

    c. Diuretics.

    d. Calcium channel blockers.

    e. Selective beta-blockers.

2-4. The first-line therapeutic intervention for mild hypertension consists of:

    a. Diuretics or beta-blockers.

    b. ACE inhibitors.

    c. Calcium channel blockers.

    d. Nonpharmacologic therapy (exercise, diet).

    e. Alpha-blockers.

2-5. Common side effects of diuretics include all of the following, EXCEPT:

    a. Hypokalemia.

    b. Hyperglycemia.

    c. Dehydration.

    d. Cold intolerance.

    e. Hyperuricemia.

Choose ONE of the following characteristic hemodynamic responses as the most appropriate for each of the groups identified in the following 6 questions.

		SYS	DYS
a.	Increased systolic and increased diastolic	↑	↑
b.	Increased systolic and decreased diastolic	↑	↓
c.	Decreased systolic and increased diastolic	↓	↑
d.	Decreased systolic and decreased diastolic	↓	↓
e.	No change in either systolic or diastolic	↔	↔

2-6. A normotensive healthy individual engaged in aerobic type exercise at 75% of predicted maximal heart rate, while exercising.

2-7. A hypertensive athlete, not on treatment, engaged in aerobic exercise at 75% of predicted maximal heart rate.

2-8. A normotensive athlete engaged in static isometric exercise such as overhead military press at 60% of one repetition maximum.

2-9. A hypertensive patient engaged in static isometric exercise such as overhead military press at 60% of one repetition maximum.

2-10. Case history:

    Male, age 18, apparently normal recreational physical activity capacity.

    Strong family history of hypertension.

    Resting heart rate of 92 bpm.

    Resting blood pressure of 138/88.

Resting cardiac output (measured at research laboratory) was moderately elevated.

At 3 minutes of Bruce treadmill protocol, heart rate was 65% of his predicted maximum.

His blood pressure response at this 3 minute interval would be:

ANSWERS

2-1. c. Myocardial infarction.

2-2. b. Increased renin production is a cause of hypertension, but it is independent of any benefits or alteration through exercise.

2-3. a. All of these drugs, with the possible exception of mild diuretics, can alter or adversely affect exercise performance, but the nonselective beta-blockers can significantly reduce heart rate and cardiac output and can have significant deleterious effects on exercise capacity.

2-4. d. Drug therapy is recommended for those who cannot or will not make life changes or do not respond when they do.

2-5. d. Watch for these biochemical electrolyte disorders in those given diuretics.

2-6. b. The normal hemodynamic response to significant aerobic exercise is to raise systolic and slightly drop diastolic pressure; this increases the volume at both ends of the stroke.

2-7. a. On the other hand, the early phases of hypertension will be noted by a failure of the diastolic pressure to drop, and it may actually rise. This can sometimes be a useful test for the deleterious effects of hypertension. The system is not as elastic as it should be.

2-8. a. The failure of the diastolic pressure to drop is easily duplicated with a static valsalva effort and should not be mistaken for an abnormal rise of diastolic pressure.

2-9. a. An isometric maneuver, especially with valsalva effort, is not a useful test of vascular elasticity, either in the apparently normal or hypertensive patient.

2-10. a. This young man, with a hyperdynamic response to exercise when challenged on the Bruce treadmill protocol (elevated pulse and blood pressure), is likely hypertensive. You would therefore expect his diastolic to rise rather than fall with exercise.

*Note that in the answers to questions 6 through 10, the key differentiating factor is the rise or fall of the diastolic pressure with exercise.

CHAPTER 3

Exercise Testing and Prescription

Brent S. E. Rich, MD, ATC

QUESTIONS

3-1. Which of the following is NOT an absolute contraindication to exercise testing?
   a. Recent significant change in the resting electrocardiography (ECG) findings suggesting infarction or other acute cardiac event.
   b. Unstable angina.
   c. Active myocarditis.
   d. Resting diastolic blood pressure >120 mmHg or resting systolic blood pressure >200 mmHg.

3-2. All of the following describe the Bruce protocol for exercise testing, EXCEPT:
   a. There are rapid increases in workload.
   b. Stage 4 is difficult because of the speed.
   c. It is better in the older/less active patient.
   d. Changes occur in both speed and grade with each level.

3-3. All of the following are components of the exercise test report, EXCEPT:
   a. The time for the heart rate to return to preexercise baseline after peak exercise.
   b. Heart rate and blood pressure response to exercise.
   c. Functional aerobic capacity.
   d. Reason for ending the test.

3-4. Which of the following is NOT an indicator for a referral to a cardiologist after an exercise treadmill test?
   a. Exercise duration less than 3 minutes.
   b. Double product <20,000.
   c. ST depression >8 minutes into recovery.
   d. Hypotensive response to exercise.

3-5. All of the following are true according to the 1995 recommendations from the Centers for Disease Control and Prevention and the American College of Sports Medicine regarding physical activity in adults, EXCEPT:
   a. Every U.S. adult should obtain 30 minutes or more of moderate-intensity exercise on most days of the week.
   b. This exercise should be done in one continuous exercise session.
   c. Flexibility and muscle strengthening activities are also important.
   d. Physical activity health benefits are proportionate to the total amount of minutes exercising or total calories expended.

3-6. A totally asymptomatic easy jogging marathoner (3.5 hours) presents for a routine preemployment examination. A mitral heart murmur is detected, and a mitral valve prolapse is detected on subsequent ultrasound. A slight delay of atrioventricular conduction (PR interval) is shown on the ECG. Your advice is:
   a. This person should cease all athletics or running.
   b. There is no need to change the exercise or running regimen.
   c. Do not run or exercise above estimated 70% maximum heart rate.
   d. Do not run or exercise above estimated 40% maximum heart rate.

ANSWERS

3-1. d. Resting diastolic >120 mmHg or systolic >200 mmHg are *relative* contraindications to exercise testing. All others are absolute contraindications.

3-2. c. The USAFSAM or modified Balke-Ware protocol is better for the less active patient. The advantage of the Bruce protocol includes the ability to test active/athletic patients because of the higher workload that can be achieved.

3-3. a. Though this may be useful information for the patient or practitioner, it is not a necessary component of the exercise test report.

3-4. b. The double product is defined as heart rate times the systolic blood pressure and is an indicator of myocardial oxygen consumption (e.g., pure 150 × systolic 150 = 22.500, which is within normal limits). A double product above 15,000 is an indicator of severe ischemic heart disease, and the patient should be referred to a cardiologist. All of the other answers are also indicators of severe heart disease and require cardiologist referral.

3-5. b. Intermittent bouts of activity (i.e., 8 to 10 minutes) to accumulate the 30 minutes of activity are acceptable.

3-6. b. Minor mitral valve prolapse is quite common, perhaps occurring in up to 20% of individuals. It does not require special attention or limitations in otherwise healthy asymptomatic persons who are not involved in intense, supermaximum effort sports.

CHAPTER **4**

Cardiac Arrhythmias in the Athlete

Steven R. Neish, MD

Steven P. Van Camp, MD, FACSM, FACC

QUESTIONS

4-1. Which of the following electrocardiographic findings is ominous and usually is treated with pacemaker implantation, regardless of symptoms?
   a. Sinus bradycardia during sleep, heart rate = 34 bpm.
   b. Type I second-degree atrioventricular block (Wenckebach).
   c. Prolonged QT interval.
   d. Type II second-degree atrioventricular block.
   e. Congenital complete atrioventricular block.

4-2. Which of the following is a normal electrocardiographic finding during exercise testing?
   a. Premature ventricular complexes, only at maximal levels of exercise.
   b. Progressive shortening of the PR interval with increasing intensity of exercise.
   c. Lengthening of the QT interval with exercise.
   d. Development of atrioventricular block during exercise.
   e. Short episodes of ventricular tachycardia during recovery.

4-3. The 26th Bethesda Conference recommended restriction from all competition in which situation?
   a. Congenital long QT interval syndrome.
   b. Atrial flutter.

c. Premature ventricular complexes.
d. Complete right bundle branch block.
e. Supraventricular tachycardia.

4-4. Which of the following is usually the most useful in evaluating the patient with syncope?
a. Tilt table testing.
b. 24-hour ambulatory electrocardiography.
c. Intracardiac electrophysiologic testing.
d. Echocardiogram.
e. History and physical examination.

4-5. Which of the following should be considered abnormal in the endurance-trained athlete?
a. Sinus bradycardia.
b. Premature ventricular complexes.
c. Mobitz type I second-degree atrioventricular block (Wenckebach).
d. Ventricular couplets.
e. Sinus pause of 1.8 seconds.

4-6. The athletic heart syndrome that is due to a physiologic adaptation to training includes:
a. First- and second-degree atrioventricular block (Wenckebach type).
b. Four chamber cardiac enlargement.
c. Sinus bradycardia and sinus arrhythmia.
d. All of above.
e. None of above.

4-7. An athlete with PVCs should be allowed to participate in all activities without any restrictions:
a. if they are asymptomatic of any cardiac type events.
b. if no structural heart disease is present.
c. if the PVCs decrease with exercise.
d. only if all of the above conditions exist.

ANSWERS

4-1. d. Type II second-degree atrioventricular block.

4-2. b. Progressive shortening of the PR interval with increasing intensity of exercise.

4-3. a. Congenital long QT interval syndrome.

4-4. e. History and physical examination.

4-5. d. Ventricular couplets.

4-6. d. All of the above.

4-7. d. Only if all of the above conditions exist.

Sudden Death in Athletes

Steven P. Van Camp, MD, FACSM, FACC

QUESTIONS

5-1. Cardiac conditions that place a young athlete at serious risk for sudden death during athletic competition include:
   a. Congenital aortic stenosis.
   b. Idiopathic long QT syndrome.
   c. Hypertrophic cardiomyopathy.
   d. All of the above.
   e. None of the above.

5-2. The murmur of hypertrophic cardiomyopathy classically:
   a. Increases in intensity with Valsalva maneuver.
   b. Decreases in intensity with Valsalva maneuver.
   c. Does not change in intensity with Valsalva maneuver.

5-3. The athletic heart syndrome, which is due to the physiologic adaptations of training, includes:
   a. First- and second-degree (Wenckebach) atrioventricular block.
   b. Four chamber cardiac enlargement.
   c. Sinus bradycardia and sinus arrhythmia.
   d. All of the above.
   e. None of the above.

5-4. The most common cause of sudden death in a young (<30 years of age) athlete is:
   a. Coronary artery disease.
   b. Congenital aortic stenosis.
   c. Hypertrophic cardiomyopathy.
   d. Marfan's syndrome.
   e. Cardiac enlargement due to the athletic heart syndrome.

5-5. Regarding an asymptomatic 50-year-old male marathoner with hypercholesterolemia, which of the following statements are true?
   a. His asymptomatic status and high level of fitness eliminate the possibility of an exercise-related sudden death.
   b. He may still be a candidate for exercise-related sudden death due to coronary artery disease.
   c. If he has a three beat salvo of ventricular tachycardia on a treadmill stress test, this finding should be considered a benign part of the athletic heart syndrome.
   d. All of the above.
   e. None of the above.

ANSWERS

5-1. d. These three conditions all are well-recognized causes of exercise-related sudden death.

5-2. a. Classically, although not invariably, the murmur of hypertrophic cardiomyopathy increases in intensity with decreased preload (and hence Valsalva maneuver), increased contractility, and decreased afterload.

5-3. d. These findings are all parts of the athletic heart syndrome, and if present in a trained athlete should not be considered indicators of pathology but rather may simply be consequences of the training process.

5-4. c. Numerous studies have documented hypertrophic cardiomyopathy to be the most common cause of sudden death in young athletes.

5-5. b. Neither a marathoner's asymptomatic status nor his high level of fitness provides absolute immunity from exercise-related sudden death. Ventricular tachycardia is not a part of the athletic heart syndrome and should not be considered a benign finding.

C H A P T E R **6**

Anemia and Blood Doping

E. Randy Eichner, MD, FACSM

QUESTIONS

6-1. The most common cause of a low hematocrit in a male endurance athlete is:
   a. Iron deficiency anemia.
   b. Footstrike hemolysis.
   c. Dilutional pseudoanemia.
   d. None of the above.

6-2. The most common cause of iron deficiency anemia among female distance runners is:
   a. Iron loss in sweat.
   b. Iron loss in urine.
   c. Gastrointestinal bleeding.
   d. Menstrual loss outstrips dietary iron supply.

6-3. Absorption of iron from the diet can be enhanced by:
   a. Eating more lean red meat.
   b. Avoiding coffee or tea with meals.
   c. Drinking orange juice with breakfast.
   d. Cooking in cast-iron skillets and pots.
   e. All of the above.

6-4. A low serum ferritin value in the absence of anemia:
    a. Impairs athletic performance.
    b. Is a common cause of overtraining.
    c. Indicates that body iron stores are low.
    d. All of the above.

6-5. Blood doping via injecting recombinant human erythropoietin (rhEPO) is:
    a. Not apt to speed endurance racing.
    b. Not a risk for thrombosis.
    c. Not difficult to detect.
    d. Not likely to go away soon.

6-6. In athletes with sickle cell trait, what is your level of concern:
    a. Any exertion above 50% estimated maximum effort should be avoided by all persons.
    b. Black athletes who are well conditioned will often unexpectedly succumb and die.
    c. Unconditioned persons, such as military recruits, who suddenly and markedly increase their physical activity level are vulnerable to the serious effects of this disorder.

6-7. A common cause of innocent stress hematuria in distance runners who appear otherwise healthy is:
    a. Shaking the kidneys.
    b. Cystitis.
    c. Bruising the posterior wall of the bladder.
    d. Haptoglobins in the urine.
    e. Ferritin loss through glomerular filtration.

6-8. Blood doping (illegal and definitely not recommended) has been accomplished by which schedule of autologous transfusions, assuming the best preservative techniques are available (e.g., response a means withdraw the blood ½ week prior to competition and reinfuse it ½ day prior to competition):

Blood Withdrawal	Reinfusion
a. ½ week prior	½ day prior to competition
b. 1 week prior	1 day prior
c. 3 weeks prior	3 days prior
d. 10 weeks prior	10 days prior
e. 20 weeks prior	20 days prior

6-9. Blood doping can be differentiated from altitude training by:
    a. Hemoglobin/hematocrit ratio.
    b. Red blood cell fragility index.
    c. Ferritin/transferrin ratio.
    d. All of the above.
    e. None of the above; the two cannot be differentiated.

ANSWERS

6-1. c. Dilutional pseudoanemia is a component of aerobic fitness. As such, it is the most common cause of a low hematocrit in male athletes, in whom iron deficiency is rare and footstrike hemolysis rarely causes anemia. The dilution is due to adaptive plasma volume expansion.

6-2. d. Iron loss in sweat and urine is too small to play a significant role. In most female distance runners, any gastrointestinal bleeding is minor and brief; although it may help drain iron stores, the most common cause of iron deficiency anemia in such athletes—as in their nonathletic peers—is insufficient bioavailable dietary iron to meet physiological needs as a result of menstrual iron loss.

6-3. e. Answers a–d outline four practical ways to increase dietary iron absorption. Red meat is rich in easily absorbed iron. Coffee and tea contain tannins that chelate grain iron and blunt its absorption. Orange juice contains vitamin C, which enhances grain iron absorption. Cooking acidic foods like tomato sauce and vegetable soup in cast-iron cookware leaches iron from the pot to the food.

6-4. c. A low ferritin value alone does not impair performance; thus it is not a cause of overtraining. It does indicate, however, that body iron stores are low.

6-5. d. Blood doping via rhEPO transfusion raises hematocrit and, to a point, can speed endurance racing. It creates a risk for thrombosis, however, because it increases blood viscosity. Unfortunately, to date it is difficult to detect. Because some athletes will do anything to win, abuse of rhEPO is not likely to end soon.

6-6. c. Sickle cell trait is more common among blacks but requires quite severe exertion, usually with considerable dehydration before the sickle cells aggregate. This is most likely in unconditioned persons who exert themselves far above their normal.

6-7. c. Runners with empty bladders will develop some hematuria. The fuller bladder has some cushioning from the urine itself, which prevents the posterior wall from colliding with the pubis.

6-8. d. It takes about 10 weeks to recover normal hemoglobin levels after blood withdrawal. Immediately after reinfusion some hematologic overload occurs and red blood cell concentration takes a few days to equalize with the plasma volume. Within 10 days, the advantages of hemoglobin and hematocrit elevation from transfusion have not been lost.

6-9. e. If a person has been carefully and serially monitored for hemoglobin, hematocrit, and plasma volume, a sudden spike in these values may be accounted for by blood doping. Such monitoring is not in current practice, however.

CHAPTER **7**

Human Immunodeficiency Virus

E. Lee Rice, DO

Murray E. Allen, MD

QUESTIONS

7-1. Acquired immune deficiency syndrome (AIDS) is caused by:
   a. HIV virus.
   b. retrovirus.
   c. lentivirus.
   d. production of reverse transcriptase.
   e. all of the above.

7-2. The immunodeficiency virus (HIV) can infect or is found in *all* of the following cells, EXCEPT:
   a. pulmonary.
   b. epidermis.
   c. male ejaculate.
   d. brain.
   e. liver.

7-3. HIV infection is:
   a. absolutely always fatal.
   b. almost always fatal.
   c. generally fatal.
   d. sometimes fatal.
   e. rarely fatal.

7-4. Concern for possible HIV infection in athletes should start chrono-
logically at:
   a. junior high school (grades 6 to 9).
   b. high school.
   c. university or college level.
   d. postcollege or at professional level.
   e. retirement of athlete.

7-5. What screening test is used for HIV detection:
   a. enzyme-linked immunosorbent assay (ELISA).
   b. Western blot.
   c. HIV serum antigen.
   d. HIV culture.
   e. nucleic acid probe.

7-6. Which of the following is *not* an "indicator" disease for AIDS:
   a. cytomegalovirus infection.
   b. herpes bronchitis.
   c. Kaposi's sarcoma.
   d. hepatitis C.
   e. *Pneumocystis carinii* infection.

7-7. Which laboratory measurement is a marker of impending serious
immunodeficiency?
   a. T helper cells.
   b. lymphocyte count.
   c. hemoglobin.
   d. gammo globulin.
   e. T suppressor cells.

7-8. The incubation period for HIV from date of contact to positive tests
is generally up to:
   a. 6 hours.
   b. 6 days.
   c. 6 weeks.
   d. 6 months.
   e. 6 years.

7-9. HIV is *not* transmitted between athletes by:
   a. saliva.
   b. tears.
   c. skin to skin rubbing.
   d. sweat.
   e. all of the above.

7-10. Which body fluid is *not* likely to be a source of HIV transmission?
   a. cerebrospinal fluid.
   b. blood.
   c. synovial fluid.
   d. breast milk.
   e. urine.

7-11. The HIV-positive athlete who has no evidence of AIDS clinically or by laboratory tests and appears healthy should:
   a. avoid all sports and exercise.
   b. avoid only competitive sports.
   c. avoid contact sports.
   d. need not avoid any sporting activities.

ANSWERS

7-1. e. AIDS is caused by an HIV virus (a retrovirus of the lentiviral type), which can insert genetic material into a cell's genes with reverse transcriptase.

7-2. b. The virus does not exist on skin surface; skin-to-skin contact is not a vehicle or source of contagion for HIV.

7-3. b. HIV infection is almost always fatal, but some rare individuals have lived over 10 years with HIV and some extremely rare cases have shown no signs of viral growth even after 10 years. It is now thought that some (very rare) individuals may actually survive HIV infection or that some variant types of HIV are not fatal.

7-4. b. Although no athlete is exempt from possible HIV infection, by high school sexual activity and drug use may start to become a problem. These are transmission sources.

7-5. a. All of these are good tests for HIV, but the ELISA is the first used and, if positive, should be confirmed by Western blot or any of the other tests. Some patients show no laboratory or clinical signs of AIDS and may require the full viral investigation regimen to confirm viral presence.

7-6. d. Hepatitis of any type is not an indicator of AIDS. However, persons with AIDS do develop hepatic illness. Nevertheless, hepatitis is very common, much more prevalent than AIDS, and much more contagious. Any disease that has previously been quite rare can be opportunistic in the presence of poor immune function and thus can be a clue to the presence of HIV infection.

7-7. a. The CD4–T helper lymphocyte count below $400/mm^3$ is a marker for impending immune system failure. Watch for opportunistic infections under these conditions. HIV invades these cells, replicates within them, and eventually overwhelms them.

7-8. d. Generally, from 2 weeks to 6 months is the duration of the viral incubation period, at which time ELISA can be positive. Delay of symptom onset (i.e., AIDS) is generally from 6 months to 10 years and maybe more for some lucky ones.

7-9. e. HIV is transmitted by contact of deep body fluids (such as blood or semen) directly with another person's internal organs (such as rectum or vagina) or direct blood contact (such as with shared infected needles). Normal body contact between athletes has not been shown to transmit AIDS.

7-10. e. Laboratory health workers handling body fluids must be careful of needle pricks of almost all deep body fluids. Urine contains low numbers of the AIDS virus but is rarely handled with needles and has not been shown to be a venue for contagion.

7-11. d. Athletes need not avoid anything if they are only HIV positive; in fact, exercise may improve the immune system. They should be careful not to bleed on another athlete's open wound. They should avoid unprotected sex with a member of either sex. Regulations about disclosure of HIV presence are inconsistent across the United States.

CHAPTER **8**

Sexually Transmitted Disease

James L. Moeller, MD

David O. Hough, MD, FACSM

QUESTIONS

8-1. The best treatment of a 15-year-old female with culture-positive *Neisseria gonorrhoeae* would be:
   a. Ceftriaxone: 250 mg IM once.
   b. Doxycycline: 100 mg PO bid × 7 days + ciprofloxacin: 500 mg PO once.
   c. Ciprofloxacin: 500 mg PO once.
   d. Erythromycin base: 500 mg PO qid × 7 days + ceftriaxone: 250 mg IM once.
   e. Ofloxacin: 400 mg PO once.

8-2. Care for the patient with suspected primary *Treponema pallidum* infection would include all of the following EXCEPT:
   a. Nontreponemal antibody test.
   b. Treponemal antibody test if nontreponemal test is positive.
   c. Treatment with benzathine penicillin G (2.4 million units IM) if test(s) is (are) positive.
   d. Followup treponemal antibody test after treatment.

8-3. Which sexually transmitted disease has been associated with the development of carcinoma:
   a. *N. gonorrhoeae.*

    b. Human papillomavirus infection.

    c. Herpes simplex virus infection.

    d. Chancroid.

8-4. All of the following sexually transmitted diseases require treatment of the patient's sexual partner, EXCEPT:

    a. *Chlamydia trachomatis.*

    b. *N. gonorrhoeae.*

    c. Human papillomavirus.

    d. *Trichomonas vaginalis.*

8-5. Possible complications of *C. trachomatis* infection include all of the following, EXCEPT:

    a. Septic arthritis.

    b. Infertility.

    c. Ophthalmia neonatorum.

    d. Ectopic pregnancy.

    e. Neonatal pneumonia.

ANSWERS

8-1. d. Treatment for *N. gonorrhoeae* should include treatment for *C. tra-chomatis* due to the high co-infection rate; therefore responses a, c, and e are incorrect. Fluoroquinolones should not be used in patients under 18 years old; therefore response b is also incorrect.

8-2. d. Nontreponemal tests are the basic starting point of the workup of a patient with suspected *T. pallidum* disease. Nontreponemal tests are only indicated if the nontreponemal test is positive. A single dose of benzathine penicillin G is the treatment of choice in this disease. Treponemal antibody tests are not used in followup since once individuals are positive, they remain positive for life.

8-3. b. Infection with human papillomavirus in females has been associated with cervical dysplasia and cervical carcinoma.

8-4. c. Sexually transmitted diseases that require simultaneous treatment of the sexual partner include infection with *C. trachomatis, N. gonorrhoeae,* or *Trichomonas vaginalis* and chancroid (if there was sexual contact within 10 days of the appearance of lesions).

8-5. a. Responses b, c, d, and e are all complications of infection with *C. trachomatis*. Septic arthritis is a complication of *N. gonorrhoeae* infection.

Infectious Disease in Athletes

Herbert G. Parris, MD

QUESTIONS

9-1. With exercise, lymphocytes show an overall:
   a. increase in number.
   b. decrease in number.
   c. decrease in function.
   d. no change.

9-2. Cardiovascular effects of fever on exercise include all of the following, EXCEPT:
   a. increased heart rate.
   b. decreased O_2 consumption.
   c. decreased blood pressure.
   d. decreased maximal workload.

9-3. A football player may return to competition ____ weeks after the onset of symptoms of infectious mononucleosis, if splenomegaly is not present.
   a. 1.
   b. 4.
   c. 8.
   d. 16.
   e. 24.

9-4. Pneumonia is most commonly caused by *Mycoplasma* in athletes <40 years of age.
   a. true.
   b. false.

9-5. Wrestlers with herpes gladiatorum may compete if area with lesions/rash is covered with a bandage.
   a. true.
   b. false.

ANSWERS

9-1. a. Studies reveal an overall increase in number and function of lym-phocytes. However, the clinical effect is transient, lasting less than 2 hours, and the clinical consequences are not known.

9-2. b. Increased O_2 consumption as well as the other hyperdynamic car-diovascular changes are affected by fever.

9-3. b. 4 weeks is the recommended time for return to contact and stren-uous activities if splenomegaly not present.

9-4. b. False. Community acquired pneumonia is most commonly caused by viruses in people aged 5-40 years.

9-5. b. False. Wrestlers suffering from herpes gladiatorum should not compete until lesions are entirely gone. The chance of a bandage coming off during competition is highly probable, leading to trans-mission of the virus to a competitor and/or the wrestling mat, a vec-tor for further infection.

CHAPTER **10**

Exercise-Induced Asthma

Robert J. Johnson, MD

Murray E. Allen, MD

QUESTIONS

10-1. Typical findings in EIA are:
   a. family history of asthma.
   b. hayfever.
   c. frequent coughs with exercise.
   d. significant fatigue at the beginning of an activity event.
   e. all of the above.

10-2. In the athlete, a key trigger of an asthmatic attack is:
   a. exercise in cold dry air.
   b. the first 8 minutes of an activity session.
   c. concomitant cold or infection.
   d. fine pollens in the air.
   e. all of the above.

10-3. The first-line medication treatment for asthma is:
   a. beta-2 agonist aerosols.
   b. theophylline.
   c. cromolyn sodium inhaler.
   d. aerosolized corticosteroids.
   e. systemic corticosteroids.

10-4. Which of the following is a banned substance but sometimes used
for asthma:
a. salbutamol.
b. fenoterol.
c. clenbuterol.
d. ephedrine.
e. all of the above.

ANSWERS

10-1. e. All of the above. EIA patients have many markers in their history that give clues to the diagnosis.

10-2. e. All of the above. There are many factors that will trigger an asthmatic attack, which vary from time to time depending on the athlete and the environment. Concurrent infections sensitize the airways, as do pollens. Cold dry air also reduces the ability of the airways to keep pace with moisturizing demands. Many athletes find that the first 8 minutes of an activity are fraught with bronchospasm, but then they find relief afterwards and can compete very successfully. Such athletes can be coached to preexercise to go through this phase of an attack prior to the actual competition. This precompetition asthmatic trigger phase may take up to ½ to ¾ hour before the remission phase is reached.

10-3. a. Beta-2 agonist sprays are the first-line approach to medicating the asthmatic. Albuterol and salbutamol are common drugs here. Use can often be limited to inhalations taken over ½ hour prior to exercise that has historically been found to trigger an attack. For the difficult asthmatic case, the other drugs can be added in a stacking manner until reasonable control is achieved.

10-4. e. All of the listed drugs are used for asthma; all are also banned substances. In Europe, clenbuterol is available and quite popular as an abused drug with ergogenic effects. For some competitions the other asthma drugs can sometimes be used with a doctor's written request and approval by the competition committee. Not all athletic boards will accept a medical letter after the fact, however. Be careful of some of the sympathomimetic amines such as ephedrine, which is banned, and which can be an ingredient of some simple over the counter cold and hayfever remedies.

CHAPTER **11**

Care of the Diabetic Athlete

James M. Moriarity, MD

QUESTIONS

11-1. Regular exercise always improves glucose control in insulin-dependent diabetic athletes.
a. True.
b. False.

11-2. Which of the following increases the release of glucose into the blood during exercise?
a. epinephrine.
b. glucagon.
c. cortisol.
d. all of the above.

11-3. Insulin is consistently absorbed at a faster rate when injected into exercising muscle.
a. True.
b. False.

11-4. Strategies to facilitate optimum glucose control during exercise include which of the following concepts:
a. exercise should be performed in the fasting state.
b. exercise may be safely undertaken with a blood glucose >250 mg/100 ml.

    c. prolonged exercise may require supplementation with glucose-containing liquids.

    d. scuba diving, rock climbing, and boxing are recommended sport activities for young diabetic athletes.

11-5. Treadmill testing in asymptomatic diabetic patients over 40 is not necessary prior to beginning an exercise program.

    a. True.

    b. False.

ANSWERS

11-1. b. False. Although exercise does improve insulin sensitivity and facilitate glucose uptake by muscle, there is no evidence that overall glucose control is improved. In answering this question, the word "always" is a clue (in medicine, "always" or "never" do not exist).

11-2. d. All three of these hormones are increased during exercise and contribute to increased glycogen breakdown and glucose synthesis.

11-3. b. False. Although studies demonstrate an increased absorption of insulin from exercising muscle, the results are neither consistent nor reproducible among patients. Patients should be treated individually and informed that absorption patterns may be altered with exercise.

11-4. c. Exercise should not begin if blood glucose is >250 mg/100 ml because of the relative lack of insulin activity. Exercise will stimulate further production and release of glucose, worsening the existing hyperglycemia. Exercising in the fasting state risks the development of hypoglycemia during exercise. Activities recommended for type I diabetes should emphasize aerobic exercise, which if prolonged may require glucose supplementation.

11-5. b. False. Patients with diabetes often do not experience classic anginal symptoms because of the presence of autonomic neuropathy. Diabetes is a strong risk factor for coronary artery disease.

CHAPTER **12**

Gastrointestinal Problems in Athletes

Jeffrey A. Housner, MD

Gary A. Green, MD, FACSM

QUESTIONS

12-1. Factors associated with increased gastrointestinal (GI) symptoms during exercise include all of the following, EXCEPT:
   a. being female.
   b. eating a large meal prior to exertion.
   c. high level of aerobic fitness.
   d. dehydration.
   e. high-intensity exercise.

12-2. Which of the following recommendations would likely be helpful in reducing GI symptoms during exercise?
   a. increasing the level of exertion rapidly.
   b. minimizing the amount of fluid intake to avoid cramping.
   c. increasing the amount of carbohydrate in replacement fluids to at least 20%.
   d. serving replacement fluids cold and with a carbohydrate concentration of less than 10%.
   e. trying to eat a solid meal 1-2 hours before exercise to induce a bowel movement prior to exercise.

12-3. All of the following statements concerning exercise-associated GI bleeding are true, EXCEPT:
  a. the site of bleeding is usually found to be in the small intestine.
  b. ischemia of the intestinal mucosa is the most likely etiology.
  c. as exercise intensity increases, the incidence of Hemoccult-positive conversion is found to increase.
  d. effective therapy may include reducing level of activity, then gradually advancing exercise intensity.
  e. large quantities of nonsteroidal antiinflammatory drugs may be a contributing factor to the development of mucosal inflammation and/or ulcers.

12-4. The rate of gastric emptying is felt to be one of the primary determinants of upper GI symptoms. Which of the following factors *accelerate* gastric emptying?
  a. dehydration.
  b. walking.
  c. a meal high in fat.
  d. a meal high in protein.
  e. catecholamines.

12-5. Based on our current understanding of intestinal motility and transit time, which of the following statements is *false?*
  a. transit through the small intestine is delayed during the luteal phase of the menstrual cycle.
  b. strength training decreases whole gut mean transit time.
  c. moderate exercise accelerates small bowel transit time.
  d. when diet is controlled in laboratory studies, moderate aerobic exercise does not significantly influence whole gut mean transit time.
  e. whole gut transit time is primarily a colonic event.

12-6. In a person with a questionable history who may have had mild blunt direct abdominal trauma within the last day to week, but who now has abdominal bloating, pain in the left upper quadrant, along with x-rays that show a right shift of the stomach shadow and a raised left diaphragm, you should seek history or laboratory evidence for possible:
  a. malaria.
  b. mononucleosis.
  c. sarcoidosis.
  d. leukemia.
  e. all of above.

ANSWERS

12-1. c. Survey studies have examined endurance athletes in terms of reported symptoms during exercise. The most commonly reported symptoms are the urge to defecate, diarrhea, heartburn, and nausea. There have also been attempts to determine risk factors for the occurrence of symptoms. It has been found that dehydration and exercising at high intensity are associated with GI symptoms. In addition, most studies reveal that women are more likely to experience symptoms than men and that untrained individuals report more symptoms. Finally, eating a large precompetition meal, as well as drinking high caloric or highly concentrated drinks, can lead to symptoms.

12-2. d. Recommendations for athletes are based on the etiology of upper GI symptoms. The most likely cause of symptoms is the development of dehydration during exercise. To avoid this, liberal amounts of fluid should be given before and during exercise. To promote gastric emptying, these fluids should be cold and have a maximum carbohydrate concentration of 10%. In patients with symptoms, reducing the level of exercise and then gradually increasing may obviate symptoms. Finally, solid meals should be avoided at least 3 hours before exercise to ensure that gastric emptying has been completed prior to exercise. It should be remembered that these are recommendations and should be adjusted for individual variations.

12-3. a. The source of exercise-associated GI bleeding is usually not found. No instances of esophageal or small intestinal bleeding have been reported. Although blood flow to the splanchnic circulation is reduced by 70% to 80% during exercise, it is quickly restored to normal levels once exercise has been completed. Return of the normal blood supply to the splanchnic circulation allows the intestinal mucosa to heal quickly. Decreased blood flow to the gut and dehydration both contribute to ischemia, which is the most likely etiology of GI bleeding. Surveys have shown a high incidence of GI bleeding with strenuous activity and vigorous exercise. Therefore advice to the athlete should include decreasing the intensity of exercise to a symptom-free level, followed by a gradual return to previous activity level. A thorough history (including over the counter medications) should be obtained from all athletes who present with GI bleeding.

12-4. b. Extensive research has been conducted on gastric emptying rate. Many studies have shown that up to exercise intensities of about 70% $Vo_{2\ max}$ (including brisk walking), gastric emptying is accelerated. Studies looking at the composition of the ingested solution have found that caloric content appears to be the primary determinant of gastric emptying rate. Other factors that decrease gastric emptying include a solid meal that is high in amino acid and fatty acid content. Although the absolute effect of hormonal influence on gastric emptying remains unknown, a higher concentration of catecholamines and endorphins has been shown to decrease gastric emptying.

12-5. c. Our current understanding of intestinal transit time is limited because of the wide variation in colonic transit and the difficulty in controlling for confounding variables. Research has shown that exercise induces a *delay* in small bowel transit time. Also, subjects who performed total body strength training exercises were found to have decreased transit times. Conflicting results have been reported in regard to physical activity and its effect on bowel transit time. However, it appears that moderate aerobic exercise does not significantly affect intestinal transit.

12-6. e. The history is typical of the blunt delayed splenic injury, but other factors can also cause splenomegaly.

CHAPTER **13**

Genitourinary Problems

Aaron L. Rubin, MD

QUESTIONS

13-1. All the following are associated with increased risk of traumatic renal injury, EXCEPT:
   a. horseshoe kidney.
   b. megaureter.
   c. exercise-induced proteinuria.
   d. malignancy.
   e. ureteropelvic junction obstruction.

13-2. The most immediate, serious, early complication of renal trauma is:
   a. hemorrhagic shock.
   b. polyuria.
   c. dysuria.
   d. infection.
   e. hypertension.

13-3. In a case of suspected testicular torsion:
   a. evaluation can be delayed up to 24 hours to see if symptoms resolve.
   b. evaluation should include surgical exploration early to salvage the testicle.
   c. diagnosis can consistently be made by using sonography.
   d. diagnosis can easily be made by using urinalysis.

13-4. Exercise-induced microscopic hematuria:
   a. has been reported in otherwise normal athletes.
   b. may be due to increased permeability of the glomerulus.
   c. may be due to other conditions, such as infection, kidney stone, or interstitial nephritis.
   d. may be investigated by repeating urinalysis 24-48 hours after the athlete abstains from exercise.
   e. all of the above.

13-5. Traumatic urethritis:
   a. is more common in female patients.
   b. may be due to saddle trauma in the bicyclist.
   c. requires antibiotic therapy.
   d. may be confused with prostatic hypertrophy due to symptoms of dysuria, pyuria, and outflow obstruction.
   e. b and d.

ANSWERS

13-1. c. Risk of renal and associated injury is increased with horseshoe kidney, megaureter, malignancy, and ureteropelvic junction obstruction. Exercise-induced proteinuria is not associated with increased risk of traumatic injury.

13-2. a. Substantial renal trauma can lead to hemorrhagic shock, which must be an early concern in these cases. Hypertension can be a late complication of renal trauma. Polyuria or anuria may occur. Dysuria or infections are not immediate complications of renal trauma.

13-3. b. Early, aggressive exploration (within 4 hours) is needed to salvage a torsioned testicle. Delay lowers chance of salvage. Urinalysis is not helpful in diagnosis. Scrotal sonography results vary between medical centers, and a high false-negative rate is common. Nuclear testicular scan is generally considered highly effective for diagnosing testicular torsion.

13-4. e. Several mechanisms have been proposed to explain exercise-induced hematuria, including increased permeability of the glomerulus and direct, minor trauma. No other cause or consequence usually exists, but other possible diagnoses must be considered in the athlete. Exercise-induced hematuria may be investigated by having the athlete avoid strenuous activity and by repeating urinalysis in 24-48 hours. Gross hematuria requires further evaluation.

13-5. e. Traumatic urethritis is more common in male patients and is seen in bicyclists whose saddle is in poor position. Symptoms are dysuria, urinary hesitancy, pyuria, and hematuria. Antibiotic therapy is not necessary unless concomitant infection is noted.

CHAPTER 14

The Geriatric Athlete

Edward D. Snell, MD

Robert J. Dimeff, MD

QUESTIONS

14-1. Which of the following changes in the musculoskeletal system is *not* associated with aging:
a. decrease in muscle mass of 15% per decade.
b. peak bone mass at 30 years of age.
c. increase in collagen cross linking.
d. decrease in collagen fiber capillarization.
e. preferential loss of type II (fast twitch) muscle fibers.

14-2. In testing the older athlete for body composition, which test is the most accurate:
a. skin fold caliper testing.
b. body weight and height tables.
c. cycle ergometry testing.
d. immersion in water.
e. lactate testing.

14-3. Which is the best way to avoid exercise-related renal complications:
a. tell the athlete to start cross-training.
b. drinking a glass of water and then urinating before the exercise or event.
c. drinking a glass of water before the exercise or event.

    d. tell the patient not to drink for at least 2-3 hours before the event.

14-4. Which of the following is an exercise-related change to the musculoskeletal system:
    a. decrease in muscle size.
    b. rhabdomyolysis.
    c. decrease in mitochondrial capacity in muscle tissue.
    d. decrease in tensile strength of collagen.
    e. decrease in bone density.

14-5. Which of the following is **not** important in the exercise prescription:
    a. determining a target heart zone.
    b. exercising at 70% $Vo_{2\,max}$.
    c. emphasizing large major muscle groups.
    d. ensuring proper and safe equipment.
    e. making sure they do not perform the Valsalva maneuver during weight training.

14-6. Weight training in the elderly:
    a. should be considered only in the robust person with previous weight training experience.
    b. should be avoided in persons with degenerative joint disease.
    c. is safe and effective for improving strength and quality of life in the elderly.
    d. is uniquely valuable for its potential for social interaction in this group.
    e. is contraindicated past age 75.

ANSWERS

14-1. a. Muscle mass decreases by 3% to 5% per decade with aging. Peak muscle mass occurs at ~30 years of age, and a preferential loss of type II fibers follows. There is an increase in collagen fiber cross-linking with a decrease in fiber bundle size, thickness, and capillarization.

14-2. d. Although skin fold caliper testing is the most widely utilized, immersion is still the most accurate. The problems in immersing an elderly person are too cumbersome to make it useful. Lactate is used to measure the endurance of muscle tissue. Cycle ergometry is used for exercise testing in the exercise prescription.

14-3. c. Hydrating the person before the event helps in preventing some of the prerenal damage that can occur. The bladder will also undergo less damage if it is not empty, especially during aerobic exercise. Cross-training may help in people with musculoskeletal injuries.

14-4. b. Rhabdomyolysis occurs with damage to sarcoplasmic reticulum, enzyme activity, and mitochondria during exercise. Fortunately, this clears relatively quickly with adequate rehydration after an event. There is an increase in the mitochondrial aerobic capacity of the muscle tissue, with an increase in muscle size through hypertrophy and conversion of type IIb to type IIa fibers. Collagen undergoes an increase in tensile strength and elasticity.

14-5. b. It is more important to find a target heart *zone* than to reach a rate. The zone is usually between 25% and 50% $Vo_{2\,max}$ and is safest to stay below 60% $Vo_{2\,max}$ in the elderly. Large muscle groups are better to target because of the increased reserve. The physician must always ensure that athletes have proper and safe equipment. It is also important to ensure that they do not perform the Valsalva maneuver during their strength training.

14-6. c. Age alone is not a factor in considering sporting activities; the contraindications for weight training in the aged are the same as in the younger athlete. Studies of octagenarians have shown excellent benefits in terms of strength and aerobic improvements with weight training. Usually the programs are low weights with high number of repetitions.

CHAPTER **15**

Dermatology
William D. Knopp, MD

15-1. When can a wrestler with herpes lesions resume wrestling?
   a. when lesions are crusted over.
   b. may not participate until all lesions are eschar free and only dry mildly erythematous lesion remains.
   c. no restriction is required.
   d. may wrestle if lesions are adequately covered.

15-2. Which one of the following is *not* a common cause of allergic common contact dermatitis?
   a. *Rhus* (poison ivy, oak, and sumac).
   b. rubber compounds.
   c. chromate and nickel compounds.
   d. mupirocin ointment.
   e. paraphenylenediamines (blue/black dyes).

15-3. What is the most effective topical treatment of impetigo?
   a. mupirocin ointment.
   b. bacitracin ointment.
   c. Neosporin ointment.
   d. betadine ointment.

15-4. What is the most effective time to treat herpes gladiatorum with acyclovir 200 mg five times a day for 5-7 days?
  a. when lesions just begin to appear.
  b. once crusting appears on the lesion.
  c. immediately on perception of prodromal symptoms such as paresthesias or burning at usual site of lesions.

15-5. Black heel can be differentiated from a nevus or a malignant melanoma in which of the following ways?
  a. punch biopsy.
  b. visual characteristic of lesion.
  c. superficial shaving of stratum corneum.
  d. location.

In the following seven questions, assume the described skin infection is in the active phase but completely covered with a dressing. Under these circumstances, can the athlete participate safely without contagious spread?

15-6. Impetigo:
  a. yes.
  b. no.

15-7. Tinea corporis:
  a. yes.
  b. no.

15-8. Molluscum contagiosum:
  a. yes.
  b. no.

15-9. Herpes zoster:
  a. yes.
  b. no.

15-10. Folliculitis:
  a. yes.
  b. no.

15-11. Herpes gladiatorum:
  a. yes.
  b. no.

15-12. Tinea versicolor:
  a. yes.
  b. no.

ANSWERS

15-1. b. May not participate until all lesions are eschar free and only dry mildly erythematous lesion remains.

15-2. d. Mupirocin ointment.

15-3. a. Mupirocin ointment.

15-4. c. Immediately on perception of prodromal symptoms such as paresthesias or burning at usual site of lesions.

15-5. c. Superficial shaving of stratum corneum.

15-6. b. No. Impetigo is highly contagious surface infection, and a covering dressing is not sufficient to prevent cross-infection, especially in any contact sport.

15-7. a. Yes. Tinea corporis is a very low contagion fungus infection, and a dry dressing to keep the skin flakes from being broken off during contact sports is usually enough to prevent cross-infection.

15-8. Yes. Mulluscum contagiosum is another pox virus condition, rarely transmitted from one athlete to another, even considering the "contagiosum" part of its name. Sexual contact is the means of transmittal, which is an activity not usually found on the playing field or court.

15-9. No. Herpes Zoster is in reality the same infective agent as for Chicken Pox, the varicella virus. Contact with the contents from under a Chicken Pox vesicle, or from open Herpes Zoster can be contagious to young children who are not immune to Chicken Pox, or to adults with immune problems, or older adults who might be susceptible to Zoster. Dry surface dressings are useful in normal circumstances to reduce Zoster spread to others, but for athletes it may not be enough. It should be noted that most young adults of contact sport age are either immune to Chicken Pox, or not old enough to suffer from Herpes Zoster.

15-10. Yes. Folliculitis is a staph or strept infection, if loculated it is a carbuncle. If properly covered, without pus exuding to the surface, an athlete can participate in sports. Some discretion may be required depending on the sport, and the likelihood of direct trauma to the folliculitis and the chance of breaking open the wound.

15-11. No. Herpes gladiatorum is the highly infectious type of herpes simplex seen among contact athletes, especially wrestlers. Covering dressings are not enough to prevent spread. Such athletes should be curtailed from contact sports untill all eschar has cleared.

15-12. Yes. Tinea versicolor is a low grade fungus infection, with almost no cross-spread. Dressing are unncessary, although sometimes used for cosmetic purposes.

CHAPTER **16**

Ear, Nose, and Throat Problems

Allen C. Felix, MD

QUESTIONS

16-1. Auricular hematoma is a common problem in sports medicine. Which one of the following statements constitutes appropriate management?
   a. the hematoma should be watched for 48-72 hours to allow reabsorption, and treatment with antiinflammatory agents should be started for pain management.
   b. aseptic aspiration of the hematoma should be done within 24 hours of injury, and compression dressing should be applied.
   c. if athlete appears 7 to 10 days after injury, incision and drainage can usually produce good results.
   d. when compression dressing is used, reexamine in 3-5 days.

16-2. Anterior epistaxis accounts for 90% of episodes of nasal bleeding. Which one of the following statements is not true for its management?
   a. when a bleeding site is identified, cautery with silver nitrate can be done and topical antibiotic ointment can then be applied.
   b. anterior epistaxis is usually controlled by direct pressure over the ala or by applying a vasoconstrictor-soaked pledget.

    c. anterior nasal packing is indicated when no specific bleeding site is identified or when bleeding is unresponsive or inaccessible to cautery.

    d. an athlete with posttraumatic anterior epistaxis whose bleeding has subsided and who has no obvious impairment or deformity requires no further followup.

16-3. Maxillofacial fractures and laryngeal trauma are uncommon in sports; nonetheless, accurate assessment and diagnosis are essential. Which one of the following statements regarding maxillofacial trauma is false?

    a. signs of facial fracture may include malocclusion, facial asymmetry of cheek, nose, or jaw, periorbital ecchymosis, epistaxis, and diplopia.

    b. facial lengthening is pathognomonic for mandibular fracture; ecchymosis on floor of mouth is pathognomonic for maxillary fracture.

    c. obliteration of the normal cartilaginous landmarks is diagnostic of laryngeal fracture.

    d. patients with maxillofacial or throat trauma must always be evaluated for airway obstruction. If the airway is obstructed, clear the airway, control bleeding, and transport the patient promptly in semiprone position after protecting the spine.

16-4. When treating an athlete with an avulsed tooth, appropriate steps include:

    a. start the athlete on analgesic agents, store the tooth in milk, and recommend follow up with an endodontist the next morning.

    b. advise the athlete to store the tooth in cold, sterile water until an appointment with a dentist can be obtained.

    c. handle the tooth by the crown, clean the root of the tooth with milk, saline, or saliva, and attempt to reimplant the tooth as soon as possible.

    d. allow the athlete to finish competing, store the tooth in saline, and recommend followup with an endodontist within 24 hours.

16-5. Which one of the following statements regarding external or middle ear problems is false?

    a. an athlete with otitis media who is receiving antibiotic agents may return to play if the athlete is afebrile, the tympanic membrane is intact, and, when the athlete is returning to water sports, the ear is not draining.

    b. maintaining normal earwax, bacterial flora, and proper ear canal acidity constitutes the best protection against otitis externa.

    c. the treatment of tympanic membrane perforation is conservative and geared toward preventing infection because most perforations heal spontaneously.

    d. Valsalva maneuver has little or no capacity to prevent barotrauma.

ANSWERS

16-1. b. The appropriate management of auricular hematoma is aseptic needle aspiration within 24 hours of injury; occasionally, incision and drainage may be required. Failure to evacuate the hematoma may lead to necrosis and fibrosis, resulting in deformation (cauliflower ear). A pressure dressing should be applied for 2-3 days after aspiration unless the hematoma was small and no reaccumulation of blood occurs in 1 hour. Daily followup is recommended to avoid pressure necrosis, infection, or allergic reaction. For athletes appearing for treatment 7-10 days after injury, debridement by a specialist is usually warranted. Nonsteroidal antiinflammatory agents and aspirin should not be given.

16-2. b. Posttraumatic epistaxis usually resolves spontaneously within several minutes. If no obvious impairment or deformity exists, no immediate treatment is indicated. The athlete should be reexamined in 1-2 days to confirm airway patency and rule out delayed septal hematoma, which may lead to necrosis and deformity.

16-3. b. Patients with maxillofacial or throat trauma must always be evaluated for airway obstruction. If obstruction exists, clear airway, control bleeding, and transport patient in semiprone position. These measures are necessary to decrease the risk of drainage and aspiration from posterior bleeding or fluid leakage. Signs of facial fracture include malocclusion, facial asymmetry of cheek, nose, or jaw, periorbital ecchymosis, epistaxis, and diplopia. Pathognomonic signs include facial lengthening with maxillary fracture, ecchymosis on the floor of the mouth in mandibular fracture, and obliteration of the normal cartilaginous landmarks in laryngeal fracture.

16-4. c. After a complete tooth avulsion, handle the tooth by the crown, clean the root of the tooth with milk, saline, or saliva, and reimplant the tooth as soon as possible. If the tooth cannot be reimplanted, transport the tooth in milk, in the buccal vestibule of the athlete, or under the athlete's tongue. If the tooth can be reimplanted within 30 minutes, the athlete has a 90% chance of retaining the tooth. The athlete should begin receiving antibiotic agents and see an endodontist as soon as possible.

16-5. d. Barotrauma, which is primarily seen in scuba divers, results from an inability to equilibrate pressure differences across the tympanic membrane. The Valsalva maneuver has been shown to help equalize pressure during descent and to decrease risk. The treatment of tympanic membrane perforation is conservative because 90% heal within 8 weeks. Maintaining normal earwax, bacterial flora, and an acidic environment in the ear canal with prophylactic drops after swimming or applying baby oil before swimming helps to prevent otitis externa. An athlete with otitis media who is receiving antibiotic agents, is afebrile, and has no tympanic membrane rupture may return to competition.

Environmental Concerns: Heat

Brent S.E. Rich, MD, ATC

QUESTIONS

17A-1. Which is most important mechanism of heat dissipation:
   a. radiation.
   b. conduction.
   c. convection.
   d. evaporation.

17A-2. The body essentially loses no heat when the temperature is approximately above ____°C (____°F) and the humidity is above ____%:
   a. 27°C (80°F), 80%.
   b. 32°C (90°F), 90%.
   c. 35°C (95°F), 90%.
   d. 32°C (90°F), 95%.

17A-3. Heat cramps are primarily related to the loss of which electrolyte?
   a. K+.
   b. Na+.
   c. Mg+.
   d. Cl-.

17A-4. What is the hallmark of heat exhaustion?
   a. increased environmental temperature.
   b. total body salt deficiency.

  c. hypovolemia.
  d. hyperthermia.

17A-5. What is the hallmark of heatstroke?
  a. increased environmental temperature.
  b. total body salt deficiency.
  c. hypovolemia.
  d. hyperthermia.

17A-6. The "critical thermal maximum" (rectal-core temperature) beyond which you must consider an athlete at serious risk of heat injury is:
  a. 39°C (102.2°F).
  b. 40°C (104.0°F).
  c. 41°C (105.8°F).
  d. 42°C (107.6°F).
  e. 43°C (109.4°F).

17A-7. You are a race physician at a summer race in Georgia. An athlete is brought in by the field team to the medic tent: pulse 165, semi-comatose, rectal temperature over 42°C, skin flushed, but not sweating very much, looks very hot and dry. What is your first step?
  a. ASA (aspirin) is all that is necessary.
  b. remove the subject to a quiet shaded place; place wet cold towels around neck and groin.
  c. a cold shower and sponge rub down with rubbing alcohol.
  d. help patient drink some very cold fluids, at least 1 L.
  e. 3-4 L of cold IV fluids immediately.

17A-8. An unusual state of shock seen in some ultramarathoners but not seen in regular marathon participants is:
  a. hypovolemia.
  b. hyperthermia.
  c. hyponatremia.
  d. hypokalemia.
  e. anaphylaxis.

ANSWERS

17A-1. d. Evaporation. Evaporation is the dominant mode of heat dissipation when the environmental temperature is greater than 35°C
(95°F). Evaporation is the conversion of liquid to gas, and requires
lots of energy for this conversion. Radiation is the transfer of heat
by electromagnetic waves, may be a source of heat gain in warmer
climates, and is the major source of heat loss during cold stress
when not sweating. Conduction is the transfer of heat from
warmer to cooler objects and accounts for only 2% of heat dissipation normally. Convection is the movement of heat away from the
body by the movement of the ambient air or water and varies with
the velocity of the surrounding wind or water.

17A-2. c. 35°C (95°F) and 90% humidity is closest to the body's surface
condition, so little exchange occurs. When the humidity is >75%,
evaporation slows and sweating becomes inefficient. When the
temperature is >35°C (95°F), heat can be lost through evaporation
provided the relative humidity is low enough to absorb the moisture.

17A-3. b. Na⁺is the primary electrolyte in sweat. Total body salt deficiency
is a reason for heat cramps. Treatment of this condition is easily
controlled by adding extra table salt to food and maintaining good
hydration both before and during the sporting activity. Salt tablets
are not indicated for heat cramps because of the high solute load
that is added to the gastrointestinal system and the irritation that
this causes.

17A-4. c. Dehydration in the form of hypovolemia is the hallmark of heat
exhaustion. The patient with heat exhaustion has a normal or
slightly elevated temperature but is usually less than 39°C. Heat
stress is caused by increased environmental temperature.

17A-5. d. Hyperthermia is an indicator of thermoregulatory failure and is
the pathophysiological hallmark of heatstroke. The core temperature is >39°C. Because there is usually (but not always) associated
volume depletion, peripheral vasoconstriction and decreased heat
transfer to the periphery result, leading to increased core temperature. This is a life-threatening condition and must be treated
quickly and efficiently.

17A-6. d. Core temperatures >39°C are considered hyperthermic, but at
42°C serious irreversible brain damage can occur, which is why it
is the critical maximum. Once seriously heat injured, an athlete
may have permanent problems in tolerating heat stress or in exercising in the heat; they may suffer easy hyperthermic episodes in
the future.

17A-7. e. This is serious critical maximum hyperthermia, dangerous heatstroke. Cool this athlete's core as fast as possible. One famous case

at the Boston marathon was treated with many (number never admitted to) ice cold IVs, and within 1/2 hour his core temperature was measured at 31°C (88°F), which is quite hypothermic. They overtreated. This was not harmful, was perhaps a little overzealous, but at least got the temperature down. This particular athlete has never been able to perform well in hot events ever since.

17A-8. c. Total body salt loss does not happen casually; it takes a very prolonged exposure to continual sweating (along with adequate fluid replacement which is required to merely continue the activity) to lose enough sodium to become critical. One typical American meal contains enough salt to prevent hyponatremia in a typical recreational athlete for up to a week.

CHAPTER **17B**

Environmental Concerns: Hypothermia and Frostbite

Murray E. Allen, MD

QUESTIONS

17B-1. The critical core temperature limit that defines hypothermia is:
   a. <37°C.
   b. <36°C.
   c. <35°C.
   d. <34°C.
   e. <33°C.

17B-2. The true incidence of hypothermia is:
   a. known.
   b. unknown.

17B-3. Most cases of hypothermia occur in:
   a. urban areas.
   b. rural areas.

17B-4. Hypothermia cases that require hospitalization only occur in the northern states in winter:
   a. true.
   b. false.

17B-5. Vigorous muscle contraction and shivering can produce extra heat production above normal resting levels by:
   a. ½ time.

b. 1 time (same as).

c. 2 times.

d. 10 times.

e. 20 times.

17B-6. "Afterdrop" refers to:

a. after the core temperature reaches 30°C, it will continue to drop.

b. during the cooling phase, when shivering stops, the core temperature drops much faster.

c. after the initial warming phase, there is a continued drop in core temperature.

17B-7. Which heat exchange system accounts for the maximum heat loss:

a. radiation.

b. conduction.

c. convection.

d. evaporation.

e. respiration.

17B-8. The "wind chill factor" increases heat loss primarily due to increases in:

a. conduction.

b. convection.

c. evaporation.

d. all of the above.

e. none of the above.

17B-9. Evaporative heat loss comes from both sweat and pulmonary loss of fluid. In average persons doing average activity, which releases more moisture to the environment?

a. sweating.

b. respiration.

17B-10. The best clothing worn next to the skin when very active outdoors during cold weather:

a. cotton.

b. wool.

c. synthetics.

d. thin leather.

e. nothing, bare skin.

17B-11. Shivering is an adaptation to hypothermia; it tries to keep the core temperature up. It is at its maximum at:

a. 37°C.

b. 35°C.

c. 33°C.

d. 31°C.

e. 29°C.

17B-12. In an athlete who will not respond to your commands by action or words and who appears profoundly apathetic, you might expect core body temperature to be about:
   a. 37°C.
   b. 35°C.
   c. 33°C.
   d. 31°C.
   e. 29°C.

17B-13. The level of hypothermia at which you would be concerned for bradycardia and arrhythmia is:
   a. 37°C.
   b. 35°C.
   c. 33°C.
   d. 31°C.
   e. 29°C.

17B-14. On a long hiking-camping trip, your buddy shows signs of hypothermia. A first approach to warm him/her up would be:
   a. undress to the near-buff and crawl into the sleeping bag together.
   b. build a fire.
   c. make a warm cup of coffee.
   d. call for a helicopter evacuation to the nearest hospital.
   e. check rectal temperature; repeat regularly to monitor changes.

17B-15. In a quite severely hypothermic person with some irregular pulse, you might try a thump on the chest:
   a. true.
   b. false.

17B-16. A common and effective method of rewarming the core in a hypothermic patient in the hospital is:
   a. cardiopulmonary bypass.
   b. warm intravenous fluids.
   c. peritoneal lavage.
   d. warmed oxygenated mist inhalant.

17B-17. Frostbite is seen first as:
   a. red flare on the cheeks or fingers.
   b. pale blanchable fingertips.
   c. white spots.
   d. black spots.
   e. blood blisters.

17B-18. Frostbite should be rubbed with snow.
   a. true.
   b. false.

17B-19. The white blisters of second-degree frostbite can be:
   a. left alone.
   b. debrided or popped.

17B-20. In fourth-degree frostbite the decision on finding the demarcation zone of healthy to mummified tissue should be:
   a. made early, even at the risk of amputating healthy bits of tissue.
   b. made late, even at the risk of letting the mummified portions hang on till they drop off.

17B-21. During a cross-country ski race on a cold winter day in Canada, you intercept an athlete with the following symptoms: appears benignly distressed, rather introverted, is still standing on the course and attempting to continue the race, albeit feebly, barely responds with slow, meaningless words, is confused and passively disoriented. What is your estimate of this athlete's core temperature?
   a. 36°C (96.8°F).
   b. 34°C (93.2°F).
   c. 32°C (89.6°F).
   d. 30°C (86.0°F).
   e. 28°C (82.4°F).

ANSWERS

17B-1. c. The basal body temperature for humans is 37°C; some persons can appear normal with no physiological adaptation responses at 36°C. However, by 35°C a person is at the limit where physiological adaptation responses become paramount. At this limit we see quite strong involuntary shivering and a voluntary effort to get warm. At 35°C there is also the initiation of peripheral vasoconstriction; the limbs become cooler to save heat for the core. At this limit, if the cold stimulus is removed, we will also see an afterdrop; the core temperatures goes lower in response to release of cold blood from the periphery as it begins to vasodilate. Below 35°C there are all the above responses, but this is now below the limit where they are initiated.

17B-2. b. Since most hypothermic responses are both common and resolved at home without resort to medical attention, there is a vast amount of it not reported. Only the major cases are recorded, and therefore the true incidence is not truly known. For those who have lived in very cold northern climates, being cold and shivering are very common but are not reported to authorities.

17B-3. a. When the weather is cold, there is no discrimination between rural or urban areas; it is just as cold. Many rural persons, because of their isolation, become more aware of the concerns for cold weather protection. Urban slums are common areas for endemic hypothermia during cold weather.

17B-4. b. Severe hypothermia including deaths have occurred in Florida. During wet cool windy days, with air temperatures only in the low 20°C (low 70°F) range, with prolonged exposure and wet clothing, there can be a pernicious depletion of body heat.

17B-5. e. Exercise that utilizes large muscles or total body shivering can produce up to 25 times more body heat production than during resting. Muscle action is a great heat producer. During warm days, we get rid of the extra heat production by sweating and a desire to lose the excess heat to the environment, but during cold days this same heat production can be saved to keep the core temperature normal.

17B-6. c. With the usual adaptive response to cold, there is vasoconstriction peripherally. During the warming phase, the first heat is often felt peripherally, which in turn stimulates vasodilation, which in turn starts to shunt cold blood back to the core. During the warming phase, we can observe an increased hypothermia or drop of core temperature, known as "afterdrop." Therefore be careful during the warming phase; a person is not out of trouble merely because warming has been initiated.

17B-7. a. The five means of heat exchange have about the following percent contribution to heat loss:

Radiation   60% (radiant loss least if curled up and insulated)

Conduction and convection   15% (major contributor being immersed)

Evaporation and respiration   25% (greatest with cold high winds, sweating more than respiration)

17B-8. b. Convection essentially blows heat away from the body surface, eliminating the very small but crucial warm dry air layer that exists next to the skin. Even when immersed in cold water, holding still will help to preserve a warm layer around the body.

17B-9. a. The act of sweating exposes a large wet surface area to evaporation, during which there is a great exchange of heat to the atmosphere when water converts to humid air (remember your physics!).

17B-10. c. Although cotton is a common and inexpensive material, it attracts moisture, which is the wrong thing to do next to the skin. Wool will also attract moisture and absorb a great deal of it, but will not lose it easily to the atmosphere. Wool will help to hold moisture away from the skin for awhile, but once wet, it will stay wet for a long time. The newer synthetic nylon and propylene derivatives will absorb sweat from the skin, and wick it to the surface, thus keeping the skin dry and insulated. Fleece-type products are becoming very popular with winter outdoorspersons. Thin leather provides almost no insulation, and of course bare skin in cold weather is ridiculous.

17B-11. b. Involuntary shivering is maximum at 35°C and below this point may actually cease. Beware of the cold person who has stopped shivering; this person has stopped adapting to the cold and without external rewarming core temperature will continue to drop, perhaps to fatal levels.

17B-12. c. Again, this is at a level with failed adaptation. The apathetic person may actually make paradoxical or maladaptive responses like removing their clothes. Their mind is confused and unable to make good choices.

17B-13. d. Now we are at a dangerous level of hypothermia. A person may look nearly comatose. Strangely enough, such persons who are totally unresponsive during the severe hypothermic phase may actually have complete memory of the event once they are warmed up. The mind keeps clicking along even if it can't respond. This can be internally very frightening for a victim, but they can't tell you their feelings.

17B-14. a. The first rewarming measure is to find some quick shelter away from the wind or rain, get the wet clothes off, and get a warm exposed body next to the victim. You want to transfer heat from the warm person to the cold person with the least amount of hindrance, and you also want to insulate them both. A sleeping bag with two persons is ideal. Others can then go about building the fire, warming some food, or preparing for evacuation. Ignore the rectal temperature; it merely exposes the hypothermic person to more cold air and won't help direct warming methods.

17B-15. b. Never jar or jostle the hypothermic person. Rough handling may precipitate ventricular fibrillation. Physically handle them very gently.

17B-16. d. All the above methods are useful for rewarming. The quickest is the warm oxygenated mist inhalant; there are a number of commercial products available that are very convenient and require very little preparation. Next in use is the warm intravenous fluids. You can warm them in the microwave or other heating device to about 42°C (108°F), or just at the level that you can hold in your hand comfortably without a burning feeling. Peritoneal lavage and cardiopulmonary bypass are reserved for the very severe cases and require a full advanced intensive care team.

17B-17. c. When outdoors in winter, watch each other for white spots on nose, ears, and cheeks; these are the first signs of frostbite. It represents actual freezing and crystallization of the tissues. When this occurs, warm affected areas immediately, sometimes simply by turning away from the wind, and holding a warm hand (anyone's) directly on the spot.

17B-18. b. Snow is cold; that is the wrong approach. Old wives' tales suggested the cold parts should be warmed very slowly. That is false; they should be warmed as fast as possible. This usually hurts, but the faster the better. When you were a child, your mother may have put your hands and feet in the open oven door at about 150°F but she would also put her own hands in too to check that you did not get overheated. This is tricky and not recommended due to the problem for heat burns. Really cold limbs can't tell how hot it is and can be easily burned. However, the method emphasizes the importance of early, quick, fast warming.

17B-19. b. Just like a friction blister or a burn blister, the cold blister can be popped and drained.

17B-20. b. Sometimes what looks like a totally lost digit is not all lost. Wait; the body will demarcate itself. This stage of cold injury requires very gentle and careful soft tissue management for infection.

17B-21. b. Note the lack of uncontrollable shivering; therefore if this athlete is cold, he is very cold, probably below 35°C. Yet the athlete is still standing and somewhat responsive, so core temperature must be above 32°C. Therefore 34°C is the best answer.

CHAPTER 17C

Environmental Concerns: Altitude Illness

Ferdy Massimino, MD, MPH

QUESTIONS

17C-1. Acute mountain sickness rarely occurs below which elevation (1 ft = 0.3048 m)?
   a. 8,000 feet (2438 m).
   b. 12,000 feet (3658 m).
   d. 20,000 feet (6096 m).
   e. 24,000 feet (7315 m).

17C-2. Acute mountain sickness is associated with all of the following, EXCEPT:
   a. intracellular edema.
   b. polycythemia.
   c. hypoxia.
   d. hypocapnia.
   e. respiratory alkalosis.

17C-3. The hallmark of acclimation to altitude is:
   a. increased heart rate.
   b. increased cerebral blood flow.
   c. increased ventilation.
   d. increased hematocrit.
   e. increased tissue extraction of oxygen.

17C-4. The single most useful sign for recognizing the progression of acute mountain sickness from mild to severe is:
   a. productive cough.
   b. heart rate of 120 bpm.
   c. ataxia.
   d. respiratory rate of 30 per minute.
   e. vomiting.

17C-5. The signs and symptoms of high-altitude pulmonary edema include all of the following, EXCEPT:
   a. pink- or red-tinged sputum.
   b. dyspnea.
   c. orthopnea.
   d. cough.
   e. all of the above.

ANSWERS

17C-1. a. 8,000 feet (2438 m). Acute mountain sickness (AMS) usually occurs above 8,000 feet. It is a benign condition and subsides in 3-4 days. AMS is the most severe when ascent to higher altitude is rapid. Of concern are the associated syndromes of high-altitude pulmonary edema (HAPE), high-altitude cerebral edema (HACE), and neurological syndromes including high-altitude retinal hemorrhage (HARH). The symptoms of AMS include headache, malaise, lassitude, anorexia, dizziness, and insomnia and in many respects mimic the typical morning after hangover feeling (which is a caution to remember when at altitude).

17C-2. b. Polycythemia. To understand AMS, one must consider the pathophysiology of acclimation. Acclimation is the process by which individuals gradually adjust to the stress of hypoxia to enhance survival and performance. At around 8,000 feet is the altitude when physiological changes begin to occur.

17C-3. c. Increased ventilation. Hyperventilation is considered the hallmark of acclimation to altitude. This hyperventilation is an attempt to maintain alveolar Po_2, is mediated by the carotid body function, and is called the hypoxic ventilatory response (HVR). Hyperventilation produces a hypocapnic alkalosis, which results in a secondary bicarbonate diuresis.

17C-4. c. Physical findings will develop if AMS worsens. Ataxia is the single most useful sign for recognizing the progression of AMS from mild to severe. As AMS progresses to cerebral edema, you may notice an individual wanting to be left alone and refusing to eat or drink. The progression from ataxia includes changes in consciousness with confusion, disorientation and impaired judgement. Coma may ensue within 24 hours from the onset of ataxia.

17C-5. e. All of the above. HAPE is the most common cause of death from high-altitude illness. It most often occurs after the second night at a new altitude. HAPE is usually characterized by an abrupt onset and typically is a noncardiogenic type of pulmonary edema. Early symptoms may be indistinguishable from AMS. The symptoms may rapidly progress from shortness of breath on exertion to orthopnea and dyspnea at rest. Early physical signs include crackles in the right middle lobe best heard in the right axilla on asculation. Pink- or red-tinged sputum may also be present.

CHAPTER **18**

The Preparticipation Examination

Robert E. Sallis, MD

QUESTIONS

18-1. Which of the following statements about the preparticipation physical examination is false?
   a. the cost effectiveness of yearly preparticipation examination has been questioned.
   b. studies show that preparticipation examination disqualifies <2% of athletes.
   c. most states do not require yearly preparticipation examinations.
   d. the preparticipation examination is a good time to counsel adolescent athletes on high-risk behavior.
   e. none of the above.

18-2. Which of the following is essential to the preparticipation examination?
   a. cardiovascular assessment.
   b. gastrointestinal assessment.
   c. musculoskeletal assessment.
   d. genitourinary assessment.
   e. a and c.

18-3. Which of the following is true of the cardiovascular assessment part of the preparticipation examination?

a. the medical history is seldom helpful in identifying cardiovascular problems.

b. exercise-related syncope may be a sign of cardiac outflow tract obstruction.

c. diastolic murmurs less than grade II are usually benign flow murmurs.

d. a murmur that increases with the Valsalva maneuver is likely to be a flow murmur.

e. b and d.

18-4. Important diagnostic tests that should be a routine part of the preparticipation examination include:

a. screening urinalysis.

b. electrocardiogram.

c. echocardiogram.

d. all of the above.

e. none of the above.

18-5. Which of the following statements regarding exercise-related sudden death is false?

a. death is most often related to a heart problem.

b. coronary artery disease is the most common cause in athletes <30 years of age.

c. family history of sudden death is an important clue.

d. aortic rupture associated with Marfan syndrome may be a cause.

e. none of the above.

ANSWERS

18-1. c. At least 35 states require yearly preparticipation examination. However, many question the cost effectiveness of yearly examination because only 0.3% to 1.3% of athletes are disqualified from sports participation as a result of problems found by examination. The examination is often an adolescent's only contact with a physician and is therefore an excellent opportunity to discuss high-risk behavior.

18-2. e. Because the stress of exercise mainly affects the cardiovascular and musculoskeletal systems, these systems are the most important areas for evaluation in the preparticipation examination.

18-3. b. A history of exercise-related syncope is probably the best indicator of an underlying cardiac outflow obstruction such as hypertrophic cardiomyopathy. Affected persons often have systolic murmurs that increase in intensity with the Valsalva maneuver (unlike flow murmurs, which decrease with the Valsalva maneuver). Flow murmurs are generally systolic murmurs, and all diastolic murmurs deserve further evaluation. The medical history is the most important tool for cardiovascular assessment and can identify between 63% and 74% of problems affecting athletes.

18-4. e. None of these tests has been shown to be cost effective as a *routine* part of the preparticipation examination.

18-5. b. Coronary artery disease is the most common cause of exercise-related sudden death in athletes >30 years of age. Structural heart problems (such as hypertrophic cardiomyopathy) are most common in athletes <30 years of age. Aortic rupture associated with Marfan syndrome is an important cause of exercise-related sudden death. All of these disorders have a familial component.

CHAPTER 19

Exercise Physiology

Peter B. Raven, PhD, FACSM

QUESTIONS

19-1. Exercise exhaustion occurs at:
   a. maximal aerobic capacity.
   b. depletion of lipid stores.
   c. ventilation threshold.
   d. depletion of glycogen stores.
   e. depletion of creatine phosphate.

19-2. In the untrained subject, which cardiovascular variable achieves a maximal value at 40% $Vo_{2\,max}$ during upright exercise?
   a. heart rate.
   b. cardiac output.
   c. stroke volume.
   d. arteriovenous oxygen difference.
   e. mean arterial pressure.

19-3. At the onset of exercise, heart rate increases because of:
   a. increased cardiac sympathetic nerve activity.
   b. withdrawal of parasympathetic nerve activity.
   c. increases in body temperature.
   d. decreases in venous return.
   e. increases in the intrinsic heart rate.

19-4. Endurance exercise training increases maximal oxygen uptake ($Vo_{2\,max}$) by increasing:
   a. maximal cardiac output, stroke volume, and arteriovenous oxygen difference.
   b. maximal heart rate.
   c. pulmonary ventilation capacity.
   d. maximal sympathetic nervous system activity.
   e. nonoxidative metabolic capacity.

19-5. Ventilatory threshold is manifested by an exponential increase in ventilation and is an index of:
   a. the maximal oxygen uptake.
   b. inadequate pulmonary ventilation.
   c. perfusion-diffusion mismatch.
   d. respiratory compensation for metabolic acidosis.
   e. the beginning of nonoxidative metabolism.

ANSWERS

19-1. d. Intramuscular glycogen stores become depleted because the intensity of the exercise exceeds the glycogen-sparing effects of lipids entering the Krebs cycle and therefore lactic acid buildup occurs in the muscle. Oxygen delivery may or may not be maximized, but there is no available glycogen for glycolysis and, with the lactic acid buildup exceeding the buffing capacity of the muscle, the contractile function of the muscle is impaired.

Maximal aerobic capacity only defines the circulation's capacity to deliver oxygen.

Depletion of lipid stores will cause the body to switch to glycogen or glucose as the substrate for energy metabolism.

Ventilation threshold is a point of increased ventilation near or at a time when lactic acid appears in the bloodstream.

Creatine phosphate is broken down at the onset of exercise and is replenished by oxidative metabolism during submaximal exercise or following a maximal exercise bout (e.g., a sprint finish).

19-2. c. In the upright position stroke volume is returned to its supine value by the effect of the muscle pump.

Heart rate, cardiac output, arteriovenous oxygen difference, and mean arterial pressure continue to increase as the workload (or intensity) of exercise increases.

19-3. b. At heart rates below 100 bpm the heart rate increase is due to parasympathetic withdrawal; at heart rates between 100 and 150 bpm the parasympathetic withdrawal continues and sympathetic activation increases; at heart rates above 150 bpm sympathetic nervous system activity increases its dominant role in further heart rate increases.

Increases in body temperature occur late in prolonged exercise and increase intrinsic heart rate, but this will not be a factor at the beginning of exercise. Also, changes in intrinsic heart rate do not affect heart rate responses to exercise.

Venous return does not decrease at the beginning of exercise because of the muscle pump effect.

19-4. a. Exercise training increases $Vo_{2\,max}$ primarily by increasing pump function, or stroke volume, at any given heart rate up to maximal heart rate. This results in an increased maximum stroke volume (50% to 100%) and therefore an increased maximal cardiac output.

In addition, arteriovenous oxygen difference (or tissue oxygen extraction) is increased approximately 10%.

Maximal heart rate, pulmonary ventilation capacity, and maximal sympathetic nerve activity are unaffected by endurance exercise training.

Nonoxidative metabolic capacity is increased by endurance exercise training, but this improvement will only help in increasing total work performance.

19-5. d. At the ventilatory threshold, CO_2 excretion at the lungs in excess of the metabolic CO_2 production occurs and therefore reflects the bicarbonate buffering of acid being produced by the exercise (Henderson-Hasselbalch equation).

Maximal oxygen uptake is defined by a plateau of oxygen uptake with increasing workload and not ventilation changes.

Inadequate ventilation would be reflective of hypoventilation and therefore an increased $Paco_2$; at the ventilatory threshold, $Paco_2$ is maintained constant while CO_2 production at the lung is increased.

Perfusion-diffusion mismatch may be present when the mean transit time of the red blood cell through the pulmonary capillary bed is too rapid (e.g., maximal exercise of a well-trained athlete); however, it will produce arterial desaturation. Furthermore, arterial and alveolar Po_2 are increased slightly at the ventilatory threshold because of the relative hyperventilation.

Nonoxidative metabolism occurs continuously throughout the rest-exercise transition and up to maximal exercise intensities.

C H A P T E R **20**

Sports Psychology

Aurelia Nattiv, MD

William Parham, PhD

QUESTIONS

20-1. Which of the following statements is *false* regarding competitive stress in youth and sports?
   a. studies have demonstrated an inverse relationship between fun and anxiety in youth sports.
   b. fear of failure is a main source of anxiety.
   c. competitive stress contributes significantly to dropout rates in youth sports.
   d. parents should emphasize "winning at all costs" to encourage future high-level performance as an adult.

20-2. Precompetition anxiety is almost always detrimental to the athlete:
   a. True.
   b. False.

20-3. Which of the following treatment approaches should be avoided in athletes with burnout?
   a. continuation of high-level athletic participation.
   b. psychotherapy.
   c. empowering the athlete as an individual.
   d. including a supportive team approach.

20-4. All the following are common responses of athletes to injury, EXCEPT:
   a. frustration.
   b. depression.
   c. anger.
   d. increased vigor.

20-5. Performance enhancement tools for the athlete include which of the following:
   a. goal setting.
   b. relaxation techniques.
   c. imagery.
   d. a and c only.
   e. all of the above.

ANSWERS

20-1. d. It is important for parents and coaches to emphasize having fun and enjoyment in youth sports. Emphasis on "winning at all costs" can contribute to a multitude of psychological problems in children, which may have life-long maladaptive psychological effects.

20-2. b. Considerable variability exists in the optimal precompetition anxiety response. Anxiety may be productive to the athlete if controlled. Successful athletes tend to perceive precompetition anxiety as desirable.

20-3. a. Rest from sport is recommended in athletes with burnout, especially in the more advanced stages. Health care providers as well as coaches should identify susceptible individuals early on and diagnose burnout before it reaches an advanced stage.

20-4. d. Coping with athletic injury can be very difficult for the athlete. Frustration, depression, anger, and decreased vigor are common experiences. Strategies for intervention are problem-focused and target-achievable goals. Minimizing uncertainty with regard to return to play options has been found to be helpful.

20-5. e. Performance enhancement skills in the athletic setting can provide athletes with cognitive, behavioral, and affective tools to execute their tasks with maximum precision and consistency. Performance enhancement is a growing area in sports psychology, which utilizes all of the above tools in addition to others.

Nutrition in Sports

Ellen J. Coleman, MA, MPH, RD

QUESTIONS

21-1. What is the primary fuel or energy source for most sports?
  a. muscle glycogen.
  b. blood glucose.
  c. amino acids.
  d. fatty acids.

21-2. How much carbohydrate is recommended to maintain adequate muscle glycogen stores during training?
  a. 5 g of carbohydrate per kg body weight.
  b. carbohydrate should supply 50% of total calories.
  c. 6-10 g of carbohydrate per kg body weight.
  d. carbohydrate should supply 70% of total calories.

21-3. The protein requirements of athletes:
  a. can be met by the recommended daily allowance (RDA) of 0.8 g/kg body weight.
  b. range from 1.2-1.7 g/kg body weight.
  c. cannot be met by the average American diet.
  d. are more important than calories to gain muscle mass.

21-4. Which statement best describes the relationship between vitamins and exercise?
  a. exercise significantly increases vitamin requirements.
  b. athletes cannot meet their vitamin requirements by eating a variety of foods each day.
  c. athletes are not at risk for vitamin deficiencies.
  d. supplementation at levels exceeding the RDA does not improve performance in well-nourished athletes.

21-5. The following hydration guidelines should be followed during heavy exercise:
  a. drink 4-8 oz every 15 minutes during exercise.
  b. drink 4-8 oz every 30 minutes during exercise.
  c. drink only when thirsty.
  d. avoid drinking prior to exercise to avoid cramping.

ANSWERS

21-1. a. Most athletes train at an exercise intensity at or about 70% of aerobic capacity, which precludes the use of fat as fuel. Also, it takes at least 20 minutes for fat to be available as fuel in the form of free fatty acids. Most athletes do not work out long enough to burn significant amounts of fat as fuel during exercise. Due to the relationship between exercise intensity and duration, muscle glycogen is the primary fuel for most sports. Blood glucose, amino acids, and fatty acids are secondary energy sumps but not primary sources.

21-2. c. Maintaining adequate muscle glycogen stores for training requires a carbohydrate-rich diet. The average American diet supplies only 5 g of carbohydrate per kg body weight, which is probably deficient for an athlete's needs. Athletes who do not consume adequate carbohydrate can experience chronic fatigue due to cumulative depletion of muscle glycogen. Carbohydrate recommendations = 6 g/kg for 1 hour of training each day, 8 g/kg for 2 hours, and at least 10 g/kg for ≥3 hours.

21-3. b. Athletes require more protein than the RDA of 0.8 g/kg, but the average American diet is quite high in protein. Resistance training promotes synthesis of contractile muscle proteins; endurance training promotes increases in hemoglobin, myoglobin, and oxidative enzymes in the muscles. Protein supplementation is unnecessary since the American diet supplies 1.4 g of protein per kg and increased caloric intake = increased protein intake. Adequate caloric intake is more important than elevated protein intake to achieve increases in muscle mass.

21-4. d. Exercise does not significantly increase vitamin requirements. Athletes can obtain adequate vitamins by eating a variety of foods each day. There is a close relationship between vitamin intake and caloric intake: the more eaten, the greater the caloric intake. Some athletes who limit their caloric intake (e.g., those concerned about extra weight affecting performance or cosmetics) may be at risk for vitamin deficiencies. Supplementation at levels exceeding the RDA does not improve performance in well-nourished athletes.

21-5. a. Adequate fluid replacement is the most frequently overlooked performance aid. During prolonged exercise in the heat, sweat losses constituting as little as 2% of the body weight impair temperature regulation and athletic performance. Inadequate intake is the primary obstacle to fluid replacement, and thirst is not an adequate guide. It is necessary to regulate fluid intake by drinking according to a schedule rather by perceived thirst. Athletes should drink 4-8 oz every 15 minutes during exercise. Drinking only every 30 minutes will result in inadequate fluid replacement.

C H A P T E R **22**

Exercise and Menstrual Function

Carol L. Otis, MD

QUESTIONS

22-1. Women with exercise-associated amenorrhea (EAA) cannot get pregnant:
    a. true.
    b. false.

22-2. Primary amenorrhea:
    a. should be worked up by age 16—no secondary sex characteristics.
    b. should be worked up by age 18—no secondary sex characteristics.
    c. is a diagnosis of exclusion.
    d. is almost always a result of athletic activity.
    e. should be worked up by age 14—no secondary sex characteristics.

22-3. Calcium needs for a young amenorrheic woman are:
    a. 800 mg/day.
    b. 1000 mg/day.
    c. 1200 mg/day.
    d. 1500 mg/day.

22-4. Which hormone values would be typical in a woman with exercise-associated amenorrhea (EAA)?
    a. high LH, low FSH, low estradiol.
    b. elevated prolactin, normal thyroid, low FSH, low LH.
    c. low or normal prolactin, low LH, low FSH, low estradiol.
    d. high progesterone, low or normal estradiol.

22-5. What disorder(s) are in the differential diagnosis for EAA?
    a. pregnancy.
    b. thyroid disorders.
    c. anorexia.
    d. polycystic ovary syndrome.
    e. prolactinoma.
    f. all of the above.
    g. a, c, e.

22-6. Prevalence of secondary amenorrhea (circle all correct answers—more than one):
    a. 1% in normal population.
    b. 100% in anorexia nervosa.
    c. 75% in trained athletes.
    d. 2% to 5% in "normal" population.
    e. 3% to 66% in athletes.

ANSWERS

22-1. b. False. Exercise induced amenorrhea is not an indication that a young woman cannot get pregnant. The focus should be in excluding other causes of amenorrhea, upon which an athlete can be reassured that pregnancy is possible once their training regime is reduced and normal menses begin. That could become a matter of timing, depending on athletic schedule and competitions.

22-2. e. If a young girl at age 14 still has primary amenorrhea, with no secondary sex characteristics, they deserve a thorough medical work-up to exclude non-athletic causes of amenorrhea.

22-3. d. Calcium needs in the amenorrheic young athlete are higher than expected, about 1500 mg/day. For example, at bony sites that are not exposed to contact or high levels of activity, they can actually develop osteoporosis, for example at the wrists in runners. Therefore, every opportunity should be taken to optimize the prevention of osteoporosis, which includes higher intake of calcium.

22-4. c. Exercise associated amenorrhea is associated with reduced level of almost all the female hormones, with the sometimes exception of prolactin. The primary source of pituitary inhibition starts from higher endorphin levels, which first inhibits LH, with secondary failure to stimulate a rise of FSH and estradiol.

22-5. f. Exercise associated amenorrhea (EAA) should be differentiated from all of the above: pregnancy, thyroid disorders, polycystic ovary syndrome, and prolactinoma.

22-6. b, d, and e. Secondary amenorrhea, among which is EAA, is seen in 100% of anorexia nervosa, in 2 to 5% of the normal population, and up to 66% in athletes depending on the intensity/duration of their sports training/competition.

CHAPTER 23

Pregnancy

Raul Artal, MD

Philip J. Buckenmeyer, PhD

Robert A. Wiswell, PhD

QUESTIONS

23-1. All of the following symptoms should be signals for a pregnant woman to stop exercise and contact her physician, EXCEPT:
   a. back pain.
   b. vaginal bleeding.
   c. faintness.
   d. increased fetal activity.
   e. generalized edema.

23-2. Which of the following exercise modes would be least safe for a woman who wishes to continue with her active life-style?
   a. scuba diving.
   b. stationary bicycling.
   c. jogging.
   d. swimming.
   e. weight lifting.

23-3. Which of the following conditions would NOT be an important factor when considering exercise for a pregnant woman?
   a. pregnancy-induced hypertension.
   b. incompetent cervix/cerclage.
   c. >35 years of age.

d. intrauterine growth retardation.
e. persistent second- or third trimester bleeding.

23-4. The primary outcome associated with exercising during pregnancy is:
a. higher probability of premature delivery.
b. increased risk of cesarean delivery.
c. lower infant birth weight.
d. greater maternal weight gain during pregnancy.
e. shorter duration of labor and delivery.

23-5. The physical examination, when evaluating a pregnant woman interested in exercise, must include the following, EXCEPT:
a. vital signs.
b. cardiopulmonary evaluation.
c. abdomen.
d. extremities.
e. all of the above.

23-6. Exercise-induced hyperthermia during pregnancy is associated with which finding:
a. The fetus contributes 25% of the increased basal metabolic rate and increased heat liberation.
b. The fetal core temperature is 0.5°C higher than that of the mother.
c. Dehydration augments exercise-induced hyperthermia.
d. Neural tube defects in newborns have *not* been associated with exercise-related hyperthermia.
e. all of the above.

ANSWERS

23-1. d. There is an approximate 50% incidence of backache during pregnancy. The appearance of low back pain during physical activity
could be a signal of several problems, which might include spasm of
the paraspinal muscles, sacroiliac dysfunction, osteitis condensans
ilii, lumbar disc displacement or herniation (rare), and meralgia
paresthetica. Low back pain is often resolved with decreased activity
and/or bed rest. A patient should consult with a physician if low
back pain occurs. Vaginal bleeding may be a sign that there is a disruption of the uteroplacental complex, which can lead to a deleterious situation for both mother and fetus. Faintness suggests a lack of
oxygen or other nutrients (e.g., glucose) to the brain. If these factors
are deficient for the mother, there is a good chance that they are
lacking for the fetus as well. Generalized edema suggests that there
is poor circulation and hence the potential for an increase in blood
pressure. Pregnant women can also develop joint effusions and secondary aching pain in the lower legs. Usually, a decrease in physical
activity and elevation of the legs to heart level will be helpful with
lower leg edema. The correct answer for this question is increased
fetal activity during exercise. This is an expected response; a decrease in fetal activity would be a concern. A decrease in fetal activity during maternal exercise may indicate a reduced blood flow to
the uterus secondary to catecholamine-induced vasoconstriction.

23-2. a. Stationary bicycling is one of the safest exercise modes for pregnant women who wish to exercise since it allows for subject control
of workload and is a non–weight-bearing activity. It is advisable to
utilize a fan to assist with heat dissipation with indoor cycling. Jogging is not an activity that should be initiated during pregnancy, but
may be continued if this mode was pursued prior to the pregnancy.
Longitudinal studies addressing jogging during pregnancy (1.5-2.5
miles/day) have not found any deleterious effects. However, special
precautions should be taken during the first trimester if nausea,
vomiting, or poor weight gain occur. During the second and third
trimester, factors such as weight gain, lower limb edema, varicose
veins, and joint laxity may make running more difficult. Swimming,
like stationary cycling, is a non–weight-bearing exercise. It is considered by many to be the safest form of exercise for pregnant
women since their changing body composition improves their buoy-
ancy for swimming. Breathing may become more difficult during
the second and third trimester. Provided that the water temperature
is not too high (above 85°-90°F), thermoregulation should not be a
problem. Weight lifting may be continued during pregnancy if pre-
cautionary measures are taken. These precautions include lifting
with light weights, avoidance of heavy resistance on weight machines and heavy free weights, and proper breathing to avoid the
Valsalva maneuver. If weight training is desired as a form of exercise

during pregnancy, lifting light weights (2-5 kg) is recommended to prevent joint and ligament injuries. Of the exercise options available, scuba diving would be the least safest exercise mode due to its potential outcomes. Potential adverse effects include decompression sickness, hyperoxia, hypercapnia, and asphyxia. Reaching the no-decompression limits presents a significant danger to the fetus.

23-3. c. Age above is *not* a contraindication for exercise during pregnancy, even for the elderly primip. However, since exertion elevates blood pressure, it is obvious that women that have a tendency toward pregnancy induced hypertension (PIH) should avoid exercises such as anaerobic or resistance exercise. Exercise may lead to early dilation and preterm labor in women with an incompetent cervix/ cerclage, and women with this condition should be warned of possible problems associated with exertion. Women who experience bleeding during the second or third trimester, a sign of possible placental rupture and or separation, should avoid any high-intensity exercise. As yet, no guidelines have been established suggesting that maternal age is a risk factor for exercise. While many of the negative outcomes associated with delivery are increased in frequency, there is no evidence that older women who exercise are at any greater risk.

23-4. c. Many people believe exercise to be a cure-all. That is, they feel that exercise will positively influence all aspects of health and/or physiological function. The data on exercise in pregnancy are inconclusive as to a positive outcome benefit, and therefore most of the studies in the literature have approached the problem by addressing the factors to make sure that exercise does not increase risks. From these studies the only scientifically supported effect of exercise on outcome is that exercising women are more likely to have lighter babies. That is not to say that there is an increased risk of intrauterine growth retardation or prematurity; it simply suggests that activity during pregnancy has some effect on reducing fetal weight gain near term. For all of the other outcome variables in this question, while intuitively one would assume that fit women would have lower occurrence of these negative outcomes, the literature does not support a definitive conclusion.

23-5. e. The vital signs of pulse, blood pressure, and breathing are factors that could be a limitation if they are outside the range of normalcy. In particular, it should be noted that at rest heart rate is normally 20% higher, arterial pressure (systolic/diastolic mmHg) is ~ 5% lower, and minute ventilation is 40% to 50% higher in pregnant compared to nonpregnant women. In terms of cardiopulmonary status, cardiac output is 30% higher, oxygen consumption is 10% to 20% higher, and there is a greater distribution of blood to the splanchnic organs. Abdominally, it is important to check for any weaknesses in the muscular wall such that carrying the fetus throughout pregnancy will not be hampered during physical activity. A close examination of the extremities will be important to determine any peripheral circulation problems. Initiating an exercise program with peripheral deficiencies can be potentially damaging in light of the risk of swelling during the course of pregnancy. In light of the importance of each of the answers cited, none of these areas of the examination can be left out.

23-6. e. Exercise has been found to have all of the above physiological features. The fetus is a contributor to the heat equation. Neural defects have not been associated with exercise, and there is an assumption that exercise is not associated with hyperthermia; however, controlled studies of significant hyperthermia have not been conducted in pregnant women.

CHAPTER 24

The Female Athlete Triad

Carol L. Otis, MD

QUESTIONS

24-1. Primary amenorrhea can be defined as:
   a. no menarche by age 14 and no secondary sex characteristics.
   b. no menarche by age 16 and no secondary sex characteristics.
   c. no menarche by age 16 but secondary sex characteristics present.
   d. a and c.

24-2. Once periodicity has been established by three spontaneous menses, secondary amenorrhea can be defined as:
   a. missing two menses in a row.
   b. missing any menses within a 6-month period.
   c. missing three menses in a row.
   d. missing any four menses in a 12-month period.
   e. missing six menses in a row.

24-3. The female athlete triad consists of:
   a. weight loss, fatigue, secondary amenorrhea.
   b. weight loss, fatigue, primary amenorrhea.
   c. disordered eating, amenorrhea, depression.
   d. disordered eating, amenorrhea, osteoporosis.
   e. fatigue, osteoporosis, weight loss.

24-4. Athletic-associated secondary amenorrhea can be caused by:
   a. hypothalamic suppression due to nutritional-psychological stress in anorexia.
   b. elevated activity–generated endorphin pulses, which inhibit gonadotropin-releasing hormone pulses to the pituitary.
   c. pituitary adenoma.
   d. anabolic steroid stacking.
   e. all of the above.

24-5. The most common cause of amenorrhea in an athlete who has previously been very regular is:
   a. anorexia nervosa.
   b. bulimia nervosa.
   c. pregnancy.
   d. excess exercise.
   e. anabolic steroid use.

24-6. Skeletal accretion (of calcium) and thus of maximum bone density is at age:
   a. 15, shortly after menarche.
   b. 25, the age of early maturity.
   c. 35, early midlife.
   d. 45, premenopause.
   e. 55, postmenopause.

24-7. Hypoestrogenemia only has adverse effects on bone density after the menopause.
   a. true.
   b. false.

24-8. The key feature of anorexia nervosa is:
   a. pathological fear of becoming fat, even when cachectic.
   b. intense desire to be very athletic; an obligatory athlete.
   c. disordered eating along with amenorrhea.

24-9. The key feature of bulimia nervosa is:
   a. intermittent dieting interspersed with overeating, plus amenorrhea.
   b. very low body weight and very low percent body fat, plus amenorrhea.
   c. recurrent episodic uncontrolled binge eating of enormous volumes of food, then purging.

24-10. The average age of menarche in elite level ballet dancers compared to the average population is:
   a. earlier onset by 2 years.
   b. same age of onset.
   c. later onset by 2 years.
   d. later onset by 4 years.
   e. later onset by 6 years.

24-11. A young married marathoner complains of infertility; she desperately wants to get pregnant. She has been training hard and steadily for the last 10 years and thinks she has a chance to place in a race 3 months hence; she wants to continue her intense training level. She had a miscarriage 4 years ago. She is in good health and has no other complaints, and recent physical and routine blood tests were normal. Her husband has a normal sperm count and morphology. What is your next step?

a. Suggest she run the next race, then take a holiday from training.

b. Book her for a diagnostic dilatation and curettage.

c. Order serum estrogen and progesterone levels.

d. Arrange for an insulin challenge test of hypothalamic and pituitary function.

e. Radiograph the sella turcica.

ANSWERS

24-1. d. Delayed menarche is the critical issue, but if secondary sex characteristics are present at age 14 then significant hormonal activity is under way and therefore primary amenorrhea is not diagnosed. However, after 2 more years, by age 16, if periods have not started despite secondary sex characteristics, then primary amenorrhea is diagnosed.

24-2. c. There are many causes for secondary amenorrhea, and merely missing a few periods or being irregular is not sufficient for labeling a situation secondary amenorrhea. Three missed in a row can be considered secondary.

24-3. d. The triad consists of disordered eating (which at its extreme includes anorexia nervosa or bulimia), amenorrhea, and osteoporosis. All of these conditions can be superimposed on a very troubled adolescent athlete who is trying to make weight, keep lean, and still perform at a time when her body is naturally trying to put on extra fat weight. Many intense female athletes can have amenorrhea without disordered eating or osteoporosis, and as such they do not have the triad.

24-4. e. There are many root causes of amenorrhea, and merely being an athlete does not exclude some of the nonathletic disorders as well. There is a fundamental difference between the athletic amenorrhea caused by activity per se (i.e., endorphin suppression of gonadotropin-releasing hormone as opposed to the general hypothalamic dysfunction seen in anorexia nervosa). One must also be alert to the fact that female athletes use anabolic steroids, but in these circumstances, they may be less likely to complain of their amenorrhea for fear of reprisals.

24-5. c. Pregnancy is still the most common cause of amenorrhea in an otherwise healthy young woman. Especially in a noncompetitive recreational athlete whose exercise dose has been steady and lacks the history of drug use or disordered eating, the obvious is to rule out pregnancy.

24-6. c. The skeleton continues adding bone mass into the third decade. From then on a natural loss of bone calcium occurs at about 1% per year. In active women this is less; in inactive women it can be more.

24-7. f. Estrogen deficiency has adverse effects on the female body at any age that it occurs and can sometimes lead to stress fractures as a marker of premature osteoporosis. Early loss of ovaries due to natural or surgical factors should be cause for alarm, and supplementation should be strongly considered unless it is contraindicated for other reasons.

24-8. a. Anorexia nervosa develops into a body image distortion, where even emaciated individuals see themselves as fat. Athletes can sometimes have body image concerns, but it is not pathological with the fear intensity of the true anorexic. Mere eating problems along with amenorrhea is not enough to be an anorexic.

24-9. c. Bulimics can be of normal weight and at times will appear normal. Sometimes they will have amenorrhea, but that is not necessary for the diagnosis. Sometimes they are quite athletic, but not always. Their body image is about normal, unlike the anorexic. But once they start to eat, they lose control and will readily identify it as out of control. They often hide their behavior and recognize its irrational nature, unlike the anorexic, who can be out of touch with reality.

24-10. c. About 2 years delay is the average for ballet dancers and other intense young athletes. This brings them up to age 14 without secondary sex characteristics or age 16 with secondary sex characteristics.

24-11. a. A somewhat undramatic but realistic approach to handling this problem is to let her complete her competition; a few more months of amenorrhea will not hurt. Once she can psychologically as well as physically take a break, if her hypothalamus is intact, menses should resume and she is probably capable of conception. If menses does not resume, a full scale endocrinologic workup might be necessary.

CHAPTER 25

Osteoporosis
Murray E. Allen, MD

QUESTIONS

25-1. Osteoporosis is associated with a deficit in quality and quantity of bone mineralization; it is:

a. a generalized metabolic-type disorder affecting **all** bones of the body evenly.

b. commonly a **patchy** disorder affecting some bones of the body more than others.

c. common in populations that are short of **fluoride** in their water supply.

d. influenced **exclusively** by the metabolic processes that occur after menopause.

e. **not** influenced by physical and metabolic considerations before menopause.

25-2. Which sport is most likely to increase bone mineral content the most:

a. no sport, suspension in a flotation chamber.

b. jogging.

c. soccer playing.

d. weight lifting.

e. swimming.

25-3. In the final definition, osteoporosis means:
   a. loss of lamellar bone.
   b. loss of cancellous bone.
   c. decreased bone mineral content.
   d. decreased bone density.
   e. fracture.

25-4. Who is at risk the most?
   a. the tall, heavy, overweight woman.
   b. the short, lean, fair woman.
   c. Negroids of any size.
   d. Orientals of any size.
   e. Caucasians of any size.

25-5. What are the critical bone mass considerations in the younger female (<30)?
   a. watch for triad problems.
   b. maintain calcium intake and regular exercise.
   c. watch for estrogen deficiency.

25-6. What are the critical bone mass considerations in the mature female (35-45)?
   a. watch for triad problems.
   b. maintain calcium intake and regular exercise.
   c. watch for estrogen deficiency.

25-7. What are the critical bone mass considerations in the older female (>50)?
   a. watch for triad problems.
   b. maintain calcium intake and regular exercise.
   c. watch for estrogen deficiency.

ANSWERS

25-1. b. Osteoporosis can be present in the inactive bone, which can be regional. For example, runners can experience osteoporosis in the wrist as measured by bone densitometry but have dense heels. Although exercise can suppress estrogens and this deficit can have an overall effect upon calcium uptake in the bones, this deleterious effect is also reduced or overridden by the positive effect of exercise itself on the bones.

25-2. d. Weight training is the sport that increases the axial load upon bones the most and for the greatest distribution throughout the body. Weight trainers have the least incidence of osteoporosis generally or at regional sites.

25-3. e. All the issues of bone calcium amounts and density are relative, and if severe enough would be called osteopenia. However, when fractures are present due to the weakened state of the bone, that is osteoporosis, a pathological state. Of women over age 60, 25% have spinal stress fractures.

25-4. b. Short, lean, fair, Northern European women are at risk. Also those who smoke, are sedentary, and lack calcium in their diet are at increased risk.

25-5. a. If anything is going to affect bone mass in the young athlete, it is the extremes of activity, perhaps the triad of amenorrhea, disordered eating, and osteoporosis.

25-6. b. The mature female is in the maintenance phase. Here one should be concerned about keeping bone mass up with regular exercise and adequate calcium intake.

25-7. c. Once menopause strikes, there is an accelerated calcium loss due to estrogen insufficiency. Although it is still important to maintain exercise and increase calcium, this may not be enough for some women who may require hormonal replacement.

CHAPTER 26

Eating Disorders

Mimi D. Johnson, MD

QUESTIONS

26-1. Who of the following is at risk for developing disordered eating patterns?
   a. a 19-year-old college tennis player.
   b. a 16-year-old cross-country athlete.
   c. a 15-year-old ballet dancer.
   d. a 12-year-old gymnast.
   e. all of the above.

26-2. Which of the following would be suggestive of disordered eating behavior in an athlete?
   a. criticism of eating patterns of others.
   b. refuses to "rest" her injuries, an "obligatory" athlete.
   c. progressive persistent increase in training regimen to "get into better shape."
   d. counts calories religiously.
   e. all of the above.

For questions 26-3 to 26-5:
A 15-year-old gymnast presents to the clinic with a 6-month history of secondary amenorrhea (menarche occurred at 12 years of age) and a 13-lb weight loss. She feels she must lose weight to compete in gymnastics. She

has added 45 minutes of stairclimber to her usual workout. She does not eat breakfast and eats only half of a bagel and a cup of soup for lunch and a salad or small amount of pasta for dinner. She does not eat meat, fat, or sweets. She admits in private that she has been binging and purging every afternoon for the last 5 weeks. She complains of cold intolerance, fatigue, and decreased ability to focus on homework.

26-3. Which physical finding would you be least likely to see in this athlete?
   a. heart rate of 50 bpm.
   b. purple hands and feet.
   c. erythematous throat.
   d. decreased fat and muscle mass.
   e. brittle hair and dry skin.

26-4. Of the following laboratory findings, which would *not* be consistent with the athlete's history?
   a. elevated urine pH.
   b. low white blood cell count.
   c. low triiodothyronine (T_3).
   d. elevated follicle-stimulating hormone (FSH).
   e. slightly low potassium.

26-5. Which next step would *not* be appropriate?
   a. electrocardiography.
   b. thyroid replacement.
   c. contract for weight gain.
   d. psychotherapy.

ANSWERS

26-1. e. All of these young athletes are at risk of eating disorders. Athletes of any sport can develop disordered eating patterns, although the expectations surrounding body image in dance, gymnastics, and long-distance running may place athletes in those sports at slightly higher risk.

26-2. e. The athlete with disordered eating behavior often criticizes the eating patterns of those around her. She experiences an abnormal amount of anxiety around injury and often refuses to decrease training to allow the injury to heal out of concern that she may gain weight. She may begin to perform aerobic exercise in addition to her routine workout and is preoccupied with food and calories. Although more common in females, the same can occur in males.

26-3. c. Bradycardia, discolored hands and feet, decreased fat and muscle mass, brittle hair and dry skin, lanugo development, and decreased core body temperature would be expected findings in this bulimic patient. Although she may have an erythematous throat immediately after vomiting, it would not typically be seen at the time of examination by a doctor.

26-4. d. This patient should have a low to normal FSH as part of a general suppression of hypothalamic function. In the presence of an elevated FSH, the test should be repeated once; if it remains elevated, further evaluation for ovarian failure should be performed. The remaining laboratory findings would not be unexpected given this patient's history.

26-5. b. The low T_3 results from decreased conversion of thyroxine (T_4) to T_3, an expected finding in a starvation state. Thyroid replacement should not be performed. Electrocardiography, contract for weight gain, and initiation of psychotherapy would all be appropriate, although not universally effective in managing this disorder.

C H A P T E R **27**

Growth and Development Concerns for Prepubescent and Adolescent Athletes

Suzanne M. Tanner, MD, FACSM

QUESTIONS

27-1. Identify an appropriate activity for a 2-year-old child.
   a. explore a safe, colorful room.
   b. play T-ball.
   c. participate in recreational league baseball.
   d. play competitive basketball.

27-2. Which of the following parameters tends to be retained the longest if a child performs the activity, stops the activity, and then resumes the activity later?
   a. aerobic capacity (endurance).
   b. anaerobic capacity.
   c. motor skills (coordination).
   d. strength.

27-3. Identify the typical time when rapid strength gains occur in a boy who lifts weights.
   a. prior to peak height velocity (i.e., growth spurt).
   b. simultaneous with peak height velocity.
   c. after peak height velocity occurs.

27-4. When does idiopathic scoliosis typically worsen?
   a. prior to puberty.
   b. during puberty.
   c. after puberty.

27-5. During puberty, what usually happens to a teenager's hematocrit?
   a. rises as puberty progresses.
   b. remains the same during puberty.
   c. declines during puberty.

27-6. In adolescent females Vo_2/kg/min max decreases; this could be due to:
   a. inadequate coaching or training regimes.
   b. social and psychological factors.
   c. hormonal changes that increase adiposity, which increases the denominator of the equation.
   d. widespread use of oral contraceptives.

ANSWERS

27-1. a. Since an infant's vision is limited (farsighted), balance is limited, and attention span is short, complex activities such as participation on teams is inappropriate. Simple activities such as exploring a room satisfy an infant's curiosity. There is no evidence that structured exercises enhance development at this age.

27-2. c. Endurance, anaerobic capacity, and strength decline rapidly after the conditioning activity is stopped at any age. Motor skills, such as riding a bicycle, tend to be retained longer.

27-3. c. It is important for sports medicine practitioners to be familiar with normal growth and development so deviations from the norm can be detected during preparticipation examinations and anticipatory guidance can be offered. Peak strength gain in a boy lifting weights typically occurs about 6 months after peak height velocity. Peak strength gain often occurs at about age 16.

27-4. b. Idiopathic scoliosis usually worsens during rapid growth, corresponding to sexual maturation stages (Tanner stages) II-IV of puberty.

27-5. a. It may be important to be aware of the typical change in hematocrit during puberty when deciding if an adolescent is anemic. A black teenage boy, for example, may experience a normal rise in hematocrit from 34.9 to 39.3 during the usual 6 years of puberty. This dilutional effect may be enhanced in teenagers who are heavily involved in endurance sports and training.

27-6. c. Even in well-trained female athletes, once body proportionality changes with increased hormone production, there is an increase in adiposity, which means that they must work harder to move the increased mass or, if they work as hard (oxygen consumption), they will achieve less results in terms of athletic performance.

C H A P T E R **28**

Nonsteroidal Antiinflammatory Drugs

Jeffrey L. Tanji, MD

Mark E. Batt, MB, BChir

QUESTIONS

28-1. Which of the following effects have been attributed to nonsteroidal antiinflammatory drugs (NSAIDs)?
a. antiinflammatory.
b. antipyretic.
c. analgesic.
d. antiplatelet.
e. all of the above.

28-2. A strong antiinflammatory and moderate analgesic effect has been most closely associated with which of the following NSAIDs?
a. ibuprofen.
b. diclofenac.
c. indomethacin.
d. acetylsalicylic acid
e. piroxicam.

28-3. All of the following side effects are associated with the use of injectable corticosteroids, EXCEPT:
a. steroid flare.
b. hematoma.
c. subcutaneous atrophy.

    d. tendon rupture.

    e. hematuria.

28-4. All of the following locations can be safely injected with a corticosteroid agent, EXCEPT:

    a. subacromial bursa.

    b. patellar tendon.

    c. extensor tendon of the elbow.

    d. pes anserinus bursa.

    e. carpal tunnel.

28-5. The best studied mechanism of action for NSAIDs is which of the
following:

    a. inhibition of cyclooxygenase, resulting in decreased prostaglandin.

    b. vasodilatation of peripheral arterioles.

    c. renin-angiotensin inhibition.

    d. the antipyretic effect of intracellular protein synthesis.

    e. inhibition of neutrophil synthesis.

28-6. Topical dimethyl sulfoxide has several side effects; the most common concern is:

    a. carrying toxic products past the skin barrier.

    b. nephrotoxicity.

    c. hepatotoxicity.

    d. cataracts.

    e. teratogenicity.

28-7. Which of the following drugs prolongs the bleeding time the most?

    a. acetylsalicylic acid (aspirin).

    b. piroxicam.

    c. ibuprofen.

    d. phenylbutazone.

    e. all of the above about equally.

ANSWERS

28-1. e. All of the above. NSAIDs have been shown to have antiinflammatory, antipyretic, analgesic, and antiplatelet properties.

28-2. c. Indomethacin is currently the strongest of the NSAIDs and has some analgesic effect as well.

28-3. Hematuria. Corticosteroids have local effects, and only in large prolonged dosages are any systemic side effects observed.

28-4. b. Patellar tendon. Note that tendons are not to be injected, but the extensor elbow tendon is not a true tendon but an aponeurosis.

28-5. a. Inhibition of cyclooxygenase, resulting in decreased prostaglandin. NSAIDs are often termed prostaglandin inhibitors. Prostaglandins in themselves have toxic effects on cell membranes and will contribute to more prostaglandin production and an inflammatory cascade.

28-6. a. Dimethyl sulfoxide passes the dermatological barrier very quickly and can carry other chemicals along with it. It also leaves an awful smell to one's breath, like rotten garlic (not good fresh garlic!).

28-7. a. ASA can increase bleeding time more than any NSAID, up to 9 days from a single tablet.

CHAPTER **29**

Banned Substances and Drugs

Wade F. Exum, MD, MBA

QUESTIONS

29-1. Problems with drug doping include:
    a. blood transfusions.
    b. manipulation of urine.
    c. administration of epitestosterone.
    d. a and b only.
    e. a, b, and c.

29-2. Banned classes of drugs include:
    a. stimulants.
    b. anabolic agents.
    c. diuretics.
    d. narcotic analgesics.
    e. all of the above.

29-3. A testosterone to epitestosterone ratio greater than _____ is considered doping.
    a. 3 : 1.
    b. 4 : 1.
    c. 5 : 1.
    d. 6 : 1.
    e. 7 : 1.

29-4. Injectable corticosteroids or local anesthetics may be administered:
a. locally only.
b. intramuscularly only.
c. locally and intramuscularly only.
d. locally and intraarticularly only.
e. locally, intramuscularly, and intraarticularly.

29-5. The recommended sanction for a second violation involving a Class II offense is:
a. maximum of 3 months suspension.
b. 2-year suspension.
c. lifetime ban.

29-6. Some biathletes and pool or snooker players take beta-blockers, because they:
a. calm the nerves.
b. slow pulse rate, allowing an opportunity to take steady unpulsed shots between beats.
c. are not banned substances.
d. act as ergogenic aids.

Use the answer key for the next questions regarding drugs in sports:
SELECT: a. if A is correct.
b. if A and B are correct.
c. if A, B, and C are correct.
d. if A, B, C, and D are correct.

29-7. When treating injuries in athletes who are competing internationally, which of the following are considered banned substances?
a. intraarticular corticosteroid injection administered immediately prior to competition.
b. intramuscular anabolic steroid injection.
c. intramuscular corticosteroid injection.
d. nonsteroidal antiinflammatory drugs.

29-8. Accurate urine tests have not been developed for which exogenous ergogenic agents:
a. recent use of synthetic human growth hormone.
b. recent use of erythrocyte reinfusion (blood doping).
c. recent use of synthetic androgenic/anabolic steroids.
d. recent use of synthetic amphetamines.

29-9. Effects generally associated with prolonged use of synthetic androgenic/anabolic steroids in athletes who are training with weights may include which of the following:
a. abnormal serum liver enzyme profiles.
b. abnormal serum lipoprotein profiles.
c. reduced sperm counts.
d. reduced protein synthetase uptake.

29-10. Use of cocaine by athletes can result in which of the following:
   a. euphoric state.
   b. central sympathetic nervous system stimulation.
   c. postwithdrawal aggression state.
   d. peripheral catecholamine uptake blockade at adrenergic nerve endings.

29-11. Use of cocaine by athletes can result in which of the following:
   a. hyperthermia.
   b. lethal cardiac arrhythmia.
   c. acute myocardial infarction.
   d. intracranial hemorrhage.

ANSWERS

29-1. e. Serious and sometimes not so serious athletes may illegally attempt to improve their performance (ergogenesis) by whatever
means possible, which might impose problems. Blood transfusions
(Class II offense), especially of another's blood, can in the immediate phase cause a transfusion reaction, and later can transmit some
very nasty diseases such as hepatitis or, less commonly, acquired
immunodeficiency syndrome. Athletes may try to fool the testing
laboratory by manipulating their urine, such as immediate precompetition catheterization of themselves and insertion of another's "safe" urine or women carrying condoms of safe urine in
their vagina. Some who take injections of testosterone as an anabolic agent will also inject epitestosterone, which will tend to
equalize the testosterone-epitestosterone ratio so that it appears
normal. All of these drug manipulations are problems.

29-2. e. Many classes of drugs are banned as unnatural ergogenic agents
or illicit drugs. Stimulants such as strychnine were among the very
first used by cyclists. Now, the amphetamines are popular stimulants that speed up reaction time and aggressiveness. Anabolic
agents such as the steroids enhance muscle bulk and strength
along with training and also enhance aggressiveness. Diuretics can
be used to reduce weight to make a certain weight class and, by
their effect in diluting the urine, can mask urine tests for other
substances. Narcotic analgesics in fact offer little performance benefit, except to induce some analgesia if one is in pain, but are definitely dangerous addictive drugs and so are banned as Class I substances.

29-3. d. Because testosterone is a natural anabolic agent, its presence as
an injected exogenous drug cannot easily be differentiated from
the natural endogenous testosterone. Also, the range of serum levels fluctuates greatly. The means of testing testosterone's exogenous addition to the body is to measure its ratio to epitestosterone.
This means the test is twofold for both agents. The ratio should be
under 6 : 1. Some athletes will also inject epitestosterone to con-
fuse the test.

29-4. d. Normally corticosteroids are banned Class III substances; as often the means of administering them are orally or intramuscularly,
these routes are banned. However, in some medical circumstances
where athletic enhancement is not planned or expected, such as
when suturing a wound, local anesthetics may be used. Also, intraarticular injection of corticosteroids to reduce an inflammatory
joint is a medically necessary therapeutic step and is not banned.
Neither of these approaches should enhance an athlete's performance above normal but in fact may help the athlete to perform
at normal without unfair advantage. Sometimes there are some

patent medications and some over-the-counter cold medications (Class III drugs) that contain amounts of sedative or stimulant drugs like ephedrine and can be inadvertently taken by an athlete for what is believed to be a simple cold. This can get the athlete in serious trouble. Absolutely all drugs of even the most simple nature should be checked closely to ensure that no banned substances are lurking in their ingredients. If in doubt, avoid that drug. However, if you plan to treat an athlete in this manner, make sure you check it out with the coach and provide the necessary documentation to confirm that such a step was fully authorized by medical authorities and the appropriate sport governing body has been informed prior to competition.

29-5. b. Class II substances refers to blood doping; 2-year suspension is used for most banned substance use offenses.

29-6. b. Beta-adrenergic blocking agents slow the heart rate, and, when a steady hand is required, a talented athlete can phase the trigger finger to release between the pulses. However, this also means a somewhat greater pulse intensity; it may be slow, but it is also quite a jolt, so the technique is tricky and can backfire. In addition, in biathlons an intense cardiac output is required to win, and beta-blockers reduce maximum output by about 10%. Some pool players still use beta-blockers.

29-7. c. Only non-steroidal anti-inflammatory drugs are not banned substances. They reduce inflammation in a pathological situation but do not add anything extra to the normal athletic performance.

29-8. b. Reliable tests have not been found for human growth hormone nor for blood doping. Blood doping cannot be separated from the higher hemoglobin found in training at altitude. However, in some athletes with very high hemoglobins and hematocrits, there can be the suspicion that they have doped, especially if serial tests were taken. However, serial testing is not part of any current testing programs.

29-9. c. The anabolic effect of androgenic steroids in fact is an increased protein synthetase uptake. Anabolic activity consists of a facilitation of protein movement from the cell membrane to the mitochondria.

29-10. d. All of the above are side effects of cocaine, a very pervasive drug.

29-11. d. Cocaine has quite widespread effects on human physiology.

CHAPTER **30**

Anabolic-Androgenic Steroids

Troy Reese, PharmD

Wade Exum, MD, MBA

QUESTIONS

30-1. Taking more than one anabolic steroid at a time is known as:
   a. cycling.
   b. stacking.
   c. plateauing.
   d. staggering.
   e. pyramiding.

30-2. _____ forms of anabolic steroids are generally associated with more side effects.
   a. Oral.
   b. Topical.
   c. Injectable.

30-3. Anticatabolic effects of anabolic steroids are due to their interaction with:
   a. blood glucose.
   b. amino acids.
   c. cortisol.
   d. growth hormone.
   e. estrogen receptor sites.

30-4. Estrogen inhibitors are sometimes used by steroid users to combat:
   a. premature male pattern baldness.
   b. hirsutism.
   c. gynecomastia.
   d. enlargement of the clitoris.
   e. testicular atrophy.

30-5. Psychological effects of steroid use include:
   a. changes in libido.
   b. "roid rage."
   c. depression.
   d. increased aggression.
   e. all of the above.

ANSWERS

30-1. b. Stacking is just like it sounds, starting with a low dose and then stacking more on the next week, and so on. It can also mean taking more than one drug at a time, often an oral and injectable simultaneously in the hopes of avoiding the side effects of high levels of only one drug. It does not work that way; anabolics stacked are essentially side effects stacked. Pyramiding is taking one drug for a week or two, then while keeping that drug at its original dose, adding another on top, essentially doubling the total dose of anabolic drugs. This can go on for up to six or more stacks, reaching a pyramid. Then when a maximum dose is reached, the stacks start coming off, actually with the first stack being dropped first, and so on, the down side of the pyramid.

30-2. a. Oral forms cause not only the systemic anabolic effects, but also gastrointestinal tract side effects as well. The oral preparations have to be taken in larger doses to be effective for their chosen purpose, and this can lead to hepatic side effects that are common but not seen as frequently with sole use of the injectable forms.

30-3. c. Metabolism is the general flux of cell activity. Anabolism is the protein buildup of a cell, and catabolism is the reduction or breakdown of cellular protein. One of the principal steroids produced by the adrenal cortex is the glucocorticoid cortisol, which stimulates the formation of glucose largely from noncarbohydrate sources and aids in glycogen storage. Cortisol also inhibits the incorporation of amino acids (protein) into muscle cells, an effect of catabolism. Anabolic steroids act as anticatabolics probably by blocking or receptor competing with cortisol, thus allowing the effect of anabolism (i.e., anticatabolic effect). Anabolic steroids also act to assist the transfer of protein materials from the cell membrane to the mitochondria, but this transfer is not initiated unless the cell is stressed; this may be why anabolic steroids do not work unless a person is in a heavy training program, which stresses their muscle cells.

30-4. c. Gynecomastia often develops in anabolic steroid users, especially shortly after they cease drug use. This often happens during the leadin time to competition when they must be clean and at which time the gynecomastia shows up. This effect may be due to an imbalance in hormone production; in the steroid use stage both estrogens and endogenous testosterone are suppressed. With exogenous anabolic cessation the endogenous testosterone does not start up that quick, but at this time the system is left without any androgen and so the estrogen production in males can progress unopposed. In addition, anabolic steroids can be converted to estradiol and estrone, which in some high dose anabolic steroid users has been measured at seven times the levels in ovulating women. This chemical castration can be permanent. The estrogenic effect can be suppressed

by the use of estrogen inhibitors such as human chorionic go-
nadotropin or tamoxifen.

30-5. e. Although anabolic androgenic steroids offer the image of sexual
prowess, they also suppress those crucial hypothalamic hormones
that are essential to a mature sexual performance. The libido is even
more suppressed when one comes off the anabolics. Sometimes the
effects of steroids will stimulate libido rage, which can be quite
grotesque. Anabolic users, especially the chronic users, can become
extremely aggressive, and can blow up in a homicidal rage with triv-
ial provocation. When they're not in a rage, they become deeply de-
pressed, especially during the withdrawal phase.

CHAPTER **31**

Illicit Drug Use in Sports
William D. Knopp, MD

QUESTIONS

31-1. Which of the amphetamines listed below has had a resurgence in its popularity in the past several years while amphetamine use in general has decreased? Most users also prefer to smoke it:
a. dextroamphetamine.
b. methamphetamine.
c. phenmetrazine.
d. methylphenidate.

31-2. Which of the following statements about cocaine is *not true?*
a. cocaine is extremely addicting.
b. the use in athletes appears to have decreased significantly.
c. although there may be some short-term benefits on athletic performance, the side effects and addiction far outweigh the transient benefits.
d. cocaine use in athletes seems to have increased significantly in the past several years.

31-3. All of the following statements are true regarding amphetamines, EXCEPT:
a. amphetamines appear to increase alertness.
b. amphetamines decrease perception of fatigue and heat stress.

    c. deaths in elite athletes using amphetamines have been caused by cardiac arrest and heat stroke.

    d. amphetamines appear to have no addicting qualities, and tolerance is not a significant problem.

31-4. The International Olympic Committee (IOC) has banned all of the following drugs, EXCEPT:

    a. amphetamines and all of their derivatives.

    b. cocaine.

    c. marijuana.

    d. all barbiturates and sedative hypnotics.

31-5. Which of the following is not a cause of death in cocaine users?

    a. intracerebral hemorrhage.

    b. coronary artery vasospasm and occlusion.

    c. cardiac dysrhythmias.

    d. respiratory depression.

ANSWERS

31-1. b. The stimulant amphetamine drugs have been used less lately by athletes, perhaps due to public pressure, bad press, and testing. However, methamphetamine has had a resurgent use with crack-smoking (cocaine), but this is not so much among athletes.

31-2. d. Cocaine is highly addictive, its use has lately increased among athletes. Its ergogenic benefits are very short-term and marginal at best, and the subsequent euphoria with aggressiveness does not enhance athletic skills. Its use among athletes is more for recreation than as an ergogenic aid. The addictive nature of this drug, and the dysfunctional states that usually follow can easily ruin a promising athletic career. The vascular and CNS toxic effects of cocaine can sometimes be fatal.

31-3. d. Amphetamines are stimulants, they increase alertness, and decrease the perception of fatigue and heat loss. As such, some athletes can become seriously heat-stroked or push their anaerobic threshold to extremes with subsequent cardiac arrest. Amphetamines are very addictive and users quickly develop tolerance, requiring higher doses; make no mistake about that.

31-4. c. Marijuana has no known benefits on athletic performance, it is not an ergogenic aid. As such, the IOC has not banned it. However, the NCAA has banned its use. Doctors should caution their athletic patients about marijuana's adverse effects upon athletic performance and skill development.

31-5. d. Cocaine has a stimulant effect upon respiratory drive; not a depressive effect like many of the hypnotics, sedatives, and analgesics. Cocaine use can lead to intracerebral hemorrhage, coronary vasospasm or occlusion, and cardiac dysrhythmias; it is a very dangerous drug, and extremely addictive.

MUSCULOSKELETAL TOPICS

C H A P T E R **32**

Anatomy and Biomechanics of the Shoulder

Todd Jorgenson, MD

QUESTIONS

32-1. What are the major stabilizers of the acromioclavicular (AC) joint?
a. the joint capsule.
b. the AC ligament.
c. the coracoclavicular ligaments (conoid and trapezoid).
d. the rotator cuff.

32-2. What is the primary static restraint to external rotation of the shoulder at 90 degrees of abduction?
a. the superior glenohumeral ligament.
b. the middle glenohumeral ligament.
c. the inferior glenohumeral ligament complex.
d. the subscapularis muscle.
e. the infraspinatus muscle.

32-3. All of the following externally rotate the humerus, EXCEPT:
a. the pectoralis major.
b. the infraspinatus.
c. the posterior fibers of the deltoid.
d. the teres major.

32-4. All of the following control scapular motion, EXCEPT:
   a. the teres major.
   b. the trapezius.
   c. the serratus anterior.
   d. the pectoralis minor.

32-5. Maximal external rotation of the shoulder occurs at the end of which phase of overhand throwing?
   a. windup.
   b. early cocking.
   c. late cocking.
   d. acceleration.
   e. followthrough.

ANSWERS

32-1. c. The coracoclavicular ligaments (conoid and trapezoid) are the most important contributors to AC joint stability. The joint capsule, articular disk, and the AC ligament are all relatively weak and provide little structural support.

32-2. c. The inferior glenohumeral ligament complex is the primary static restraint to external rotation while the arm is 90 degrees abducted. Overhand throwing requires abduction with external rotation (often extreme), a position in which the shoulder is extremely vulnerable to anterior subluxation/dislocation. Loss of integrity of the inferior glenohumeral ligament complex is a major cause of anterior glenohumeral instability in throwing athletes.

32-3. a. The pectoralis major inserts on the crest of the greater tubercle of the humerus and, therefore, cannot externally rotate the humerus.

32-4. a. The teres major, originating on the inferior angle of the scapula and inserting on the crest of the lesser tubercle of the humerus, acts on the glenohumeral joint. The trapezius, serratus anterior, and pectoralis minor all originate on the axial skeleton and insert on the scapula.

32-5. c. The shoulder is maximally externally rotated at the end of the late cocking phase of throwing, just before acceleration begins.

CHAPTER **33**

History and Physical Examination of the Shoulder

Greg Hoeksema, MD

QUESTIONS

33-1. A recreational weight lifter with no history of trauma has been lifting three times a week for 8 years. Over the past several months, he has noted an insidious onset of pain in the anterior aspect of his shoulder. Originally, the pain improved with relative rest and some aspirin, but every time he returns to lifting the pain recurs. He also notes that recently he gets a well-localized sharp pain when he reaches across his body to part his hair. There is no pain at rest, but he has a grinding sensation even with passive arm motion. His most likely diagnosis is:
   a. glenohumeral instability.
   b. impingement syndrome.
   c. rotator cuff tear.
   d. acromioclavicular joint arthrosis/arthritis.

33-2. A young female volleyball player who works as a stocker in the local grocery store complains of insidious onset of pain in her dominant shoulder. Originally, the pain occurred just while playing volleyball and would get better with rest. Now, however, she is no longer able to play because of the pain. Instead, she has tried to lift weights to stay fit, but all overhead lifts like the military press cause pain. She has also had problems at work when she is stocking the upper shelves. It has gotten to the point where her shoulder aches all the time and even wakes her from sleep, especially if she sleeps on her side. She cannot even wash her hair without causing pain. Rest from sports, daily icing, and aspirin have only provided minimal relief. Her most likely diagnosis is:

a. glenohumeral instability.
b. impingement syndrome.
c. rotator cuff tear.
d. acromioclavicular joint arthrosis/arthritis.

33-3. An elderly man who walks daily tripped on the stairs 2 weeks ago but was able to grab the handrail to prevent a fall; however, in doing so, he noted a sharp pain in his shoulder. Since then, he has noted an improvement in the pain, which seems to be mostly on the top of his shoulder joint. He notes that he is having difficulty lifting objects at home like a gallon jug of milk. He also states that he has to help lift his arm with his other hand to get it up to his head to wash his hair. His most likely diagnosis is:

a. glenohumeral instability.
b. impingement syndrome.
c. rotator cuff tear.
d. acromioclavicular joint arthrosis/arthritis.

33-4. Which of the following would be important components of the physical examination of the elderly patient in the above question?

a. observe him as he removes his shirt for the examination.
b. drop test for supraspinatus strength.
c. load-shift test for glenohumeral stability.
d. palpation of the acromioclavicular joint.
e. all of the above.

33-5. All of the following may be found in a right-handed college tennis player who continues to practice despite a known history of chronic impingement syndrome, EXCEPT:

a. positive impingement sign.
b. apparent asymmetry with the right shoulder carried lower than the left.
c. supraspinatus atrophy.
d. positive drop test.
e. grade I anterior subluxation.

ANSWERS

33-1. d. Acromioclavicular arthrosis/arthritis. The history of insidious onset of a well-localized pain in the anterior aspect of the shoulder, especially with cross-body adduction, is typical of acromioclavicular
joint pathology, especially in a long-term weight lifter. The grinding
sensation is a nonspecific complaint that in this case is likely the result of the degeneration of the acromioclavicular joint disc. There is
no history of trauma to support a diagnosis of glenohumeral instability. Although this patient is at risk of developing impingement
syndrome, the history of a well-localized, sharp pain is not consistent. Additionally, pain with overhead activities (vs. cross-body
adduction) is more typical of impingement syndrome. An actual rotator cuff tear would likely result in more significant functional
disability. In addition, repetitive strain on the acromioclavicular
joint may lead to distal clavicular avascular necrosis and collapse.
Anabolic steroid use can also be a factor in aseptic necrosis.

33-2. b. Impingement syndrome. This is a classic history of supraspinatus
tendinitis with the typical insidious onset of poorly localized aching
shoulder pain in an overhead athlete, progression of symptoms to
interfere with activities of daily living, and nocturnal pain that
wakes her from sleep. There is no history of trauma to support a diagnosis of glenohumeral instability, although subtle glenohumeral
subluxation maybe the actual primary pathology that has led to development of secondary impingement syndrome. Rotator cuff tear
would likely result in more significant disability and would be unusual in a young patient. Acromioclavicular joint pathology is described in the previous answer.

33-3. c. Rotator cuff tear. Although unusual in young athletes, actual rotator cuff tears are not uncommon in the elderly and can appear almost spontaneously. The history of significant functional disability
with inability to effectively fully abduct the arm is relatively specific
for rotator cuff tear. Impingement syndrome may cause pain with
abduction but should not result in inability to abduct the arm. Although it is possible to sustain a rotator cuff tear in a glenohumeral
dislocation in the elderly, the history of the original injury does not
support this diagnosis. Also, a traumatic acromioclavicular separation usually results from a downward force from the superior aspect
of the shoulder and should not result in inability to abduct the arm.
Impingement syndrome does not result from a single traumatic
episode.

33-4. e. All of the above. Any patient with complaint of shoulder pain or
disability should have a thorough examination of all components of
the shoulder girdle complex. Very useful information can be gleaned
by watching the patient undress; level of functional disability can be

assessed. In this patient the drop test is a specific test for presence of rotator cuff tear. See also discussion above in the previous answer.

33-5. d. Positive drop test. This test is most consistent with the presence of a significant rotator cuff tear, and it is unlikely that an athlete could continue to play tennis with an actual tear. However, this patient is at risk of developing an attritional tear. Certainly, the impingement sign would be positive. Because the condition is chronic, supraspinatus atrophy may be present. It is also common to find subtle glenohumeral subluxation in a young patient with impingement syndrome. Commonly, patients normally will carry their dominant shoulder lower than their nondominant shoulder.

CHAPTER **34**

Impingement Syndrome and Rotator Cuff Injuries

Anthony J. Saglimbeni, MD

David E. J. Bazzo, MD

QUESTIONS

34-1. What is the primary external rotator of the shoulder?
   a. subscapularis.
   b. infraspinatus.
   c. supraspinatus.
   d. deltoid.
   e. pectoralis major.

34-2. Impingement syndrome of the shoulder is the result of the:
   a. deltoid muscle compressing the bursa, causing pain.
   b. humeral head slipping from the glenoid fossa, causing pain.
   c. supraspinatus tendon becoming pinched between the humeral head and the coracoacromial arch.
   d. biceps tendon becoming pinched between the humeral head and the acromion.
   e. subscapularis tendon becoming pinched between the neck of the humerus and the glenoid.

34-3. A young baseball pitcher presents with shoulder impingement; what is the most likely etiology?
   a. underdeveloped muscles of the rotator cuff, causing gleno-humeral instability.

b. a Bigliani type III acromion.
c. acromioclavicular arthritis with subacromial spur.
d. calcific tendinitis.
e. osteochondritis dissecans.

34-4. What is the most common *acute* shoulder injury in throwing sports?
a. supraspinatus tendinitis.
b. rotator cuff tear.
c. anterior glenohumeral dislocation.
d. acromioclavicular separation.
e. biceps tendinitis.

34-5. Which of the following is *not* considered an articulation of the shoulder?
a. glenohumeral.
b. acromioclavicular.
c. sternoclavicular.
d. scapulothoracic.
e. coracoacromial.

34-6. A rotator cuff tear associated with abductor dysfunction is best treated with:
a. rest, ice, and nonsteroidal antiinflammatory drugs.
b. physical therapy consisting of range of motion and strengthening.
c. corticosteroid injection.
d. surgical repair.
e. immobilization with arm sling.

34-7. A 22-year-old right-handed professional sand volleyball player presents with insidious onset of right shoulder pain. He states that he is no longer effective in spiking the ball secondary to pain. Physical examination reveals a well-musculatured thin male with no obvious shoulder asymmetry. There is tenderness to palpation at the right anterolateral shoulder. Passive elevation is limited, secondary to pain. Internal and external rotation is preserved. Distal neurovasculature is intact. Instability tests are negative. The initial treatment would include all of the following, EXCEPT:
a. relative rest, ice, and nonsteroidal antiinflammatory drugs.
b. range of motion followed by strengthening exercises.
c. surgical decompression.
d. cross-training.

34-8. In *acute* rotator cuff tears all of the following evaluations *can* be positive, EXCEPT:
a. physical examination.
b. plain films.
c. magnetic resonance imaging.
d. arthrography.
e. arthroscopy.

34-9. In throwing sports, what is the most common shoulder injury?
   a. dislocation of the glenohumeral joint.
   b. supraspinatus tendinitis.
   c. acromioclavicular joint subluxation.
   d. subluxation or inflammation of the biceps tendon.
   e. anterior labrum tear.

34-10. In elite swimmers with impingement syndrome the stroke that is typically most painful is the:
   a. backstroke.
   b. breaststroke.
   c. crawl.
   d. butterfly.

34-11. In the above question on shoulder impingement the "swimming" reason for the impingement is:
   a. the forward reach is too far.
   b. more range of extension and abduction needed to clear the water.
   c. the downwards and backwards sweep past the body stretches the supraspinatus.
   d. extrainternal humeral rotation during flexion.

ANSWERS

34-1. b. The four muscles that comprise the rotator cuff are the supraspinatus, infraspinatus, teres minor, and subscapularis. The supraspinatus is responsible for elevation. The infraspinatus and teres minor are responsible for external rotation. The subscapularis is responsible for internal rotation. All of these muscles also assist in the dynamic stabilization of the shoulder joint.

34-2. c. In impingement syndrome either the supraspinatus muscle becomes too large for the subacromial space through which it passes or the space is too small. The supraspinatus tendon increases in size secondary to muscle hypertrophy, inflammation/edema, and fibrosis. The decrease in space can be secondary to a beaked or curved shape to the posterior leading edge of the acromion, arthritis (osteophyte formation), chronic fibrositis, or genetic predisposition. The other answers above can be a source of shoulder pain but not of the impingement type.

34-3. a. The key to this question is that this is a young player. This refers to the secondary extrinsic mechanism of impingement syndrome, with a functional loss of subacromial space secondary to glenohumeral joint instability. All of the other answers (except for e, osteochondritis dissecans) are mechanisms of impingement but occur in older persons and generally are not commonly seen in young athletes.

34-4. b. Rotator cuff injuries are the most common *acute* shoulder injury in throwing sports. All of the rotator cuff tendons pass through a limited space and are subject to mechanical friction. Therefore, with overuse and subsequent inflammation, pain and hence injury occur. Acromioclavicular separation and glenohumeral dislocation also are acute injuries but are less common. The tendinitis problems are not commonly acute. High-risk sports include all throwing sports, swimming, tennis, volleyball, and weight lifting. Nonthrowing/overhead sports have a different occurrence of acute shoulder injuries.

34-5. e. The coracoacromial is not an articulation. There is a ligament connecting these two parts of the scapula (one bone), but the functional significance of this structure is unknown. It has been postulated that this ligament is an evolutional remnant from our quadruped days, and may be a vestigial continuation of the short biceps muscle.

34-6. d. The above finding is indicative of a complete rotator cuff tear. Referral to an orthopedic surgeon for surgical repair of the defect will give optimal treatment results. Incomplete tears with preservation of most function should get a trial of conservative treatment with relative rest (evidence of repeat strains), ice, nonsteroidal antiinflammatory drugs, range of motion, and progressive strengthening.

34-7. c. The key word is *initial* treatment. Surgical decompression is considered only when conservative therapy has failed for treatment of impingement syndrome, which is the correct diagnosis for the above volleyball player. All of the other modalities are included in conservative management. Impingement syndrome, as opposed to complete rotator cuff tear, necessitates initial conservative treatment. Surgical therapy is reserved for recalcitrant cases.

34-8. b. Plain films are normal in *acute* rotator cuff tears. In complete *chronic* rotator cuff tears, plain films may show the humerus superiorly displaced.

34-9. b. Supraspinatus tendinitis is the most common shoulder injury in sports, and in throwing sports even the acute tear of the supraspinatus is common.

34-10. d. The butterfly does not allow any compensatory motions to protect the supraspinatus and must be performed with both arms simultaneously hyperabducted through a full range of extension to flexion. The other swim strokes allow for some rotation of the trunk, which reduces the extent of the abduction.

34-11. b. The full range of the extension during abduction can wring out the supraspinatus and pinch it under the acromion.

CHAPTER 35

Shoulder Instability

Thomas J. Gill, MD

Lyle J. Micheli, MD

QUESTIONS

35-1. What is the most important restraint to anterior dislocation of the humeral head?
   a. glenoid.
   b. glenoid labrum.
   c. subscapularis.
   d. inferior glenohumeral ligament complex.
   e. middle glenohumeral ligament.

35-2. The position of maximal anterior instability of the shoulder comprises:
   a. adduction, internal rotation, flexion.
   b. adduction, external rotation, extension.
   c. abduction, internal rotation, flexion.
   d. abduction, external rotation, extension.
   e. abduction, external rotation, flexion.

35-3. The most common site of dislocation of the humeral head is:
   a. posterior.
   b. subcoracoid.
   c. subclavicular.
   d. intrathoracic.
   e. inferior.

35-4. The most common symptom in a patient with instability of the shoulder is:
   a. clicking.
   b. sense of shoulder "popping out."
   c. weakness.
   d. numbness.
   e. pain.

35-5. The most sensitive physical finding in a patient with instability is:
   a. impingement.
   b. sulcus sign.
   c. apprehension sign.
   d. decreased external rotation.
   e. load test.

35-6. A cyclist falls off the bike and lands upside down on the top of the shoulder. The arm was not extended. She presents with moderate pain, maybe a day or two later. Your suspected clinical diagnosis is most likely:
   a. anterior glenohumeral dislocation.
   b. posterior glenohumeral dislocation.
   c. acromioclavicular separation.
   d. rotator cuff tear.
   e. brachial plexus injury.

35-7. A football player reaches out laterally to attempt an arm tackle. The arm is forced into abduction and external rotation. He comes off the field with severe pain and inability to move the shoulder. The likely diagnosis is:
   a. anterior glenohumeral dislocation.
   b. posterior glenohumeral dislocation.
   c. acromioclavicular separation.
   d. rotator cuff tear.
   e. brachial plexus injury.

35-8. A stress fracture of the coracoid process is most common in which group of athletes:
   a. swimmers.
   b. baseball pitchers.
   c. tennis players.
   d. trapshooters.
   e. rowers.

ANSWERS

35-1. d. The glenoid can only resist direct forces due to its unconstrained anatomy. The fibrocartilaginous labrum increases the radius of curvature of the glenoid socket and provides added resistance to humeral head subluxation. The subscapularis is a dynamic stabilizer that is an important secondary restraint to anterior dislocation, while the middle glenohumeral ligament is a static stabilizer that also functions as a secondary restraint. Selective cutting experiments have shown the inferior glenohumeral ligament complex to be the primary restraint to anterior dislocation of the humeral head. When it is pulled off the glenoid with the labrum, it is referred to as the Bankart lesion.

35-2. d. Abduction, external rotation, and extension minimize glenohumeral contact and rely on the static and dynamic shoulder stabilizers for preventing dislocation. This is the position in which the upper extremity is placed for the "apprehension test." This is also the cocking position during baseball pitching. Adduction, internal rotation, and flexion represent the position of posterior instability.

35-3. b. Anterior dislocations account for 95% of all shoulder dislocations. Pure inferior dislocations (luxatio erecta) are extremely rare. Posterior dislocations are most commonly seen after a direct anterior blow, seizures, or electric shock or in alcoholics.

35-4. e. Pain is the most common symptom of shoulder instability. The remaining choices may also be present.

35-5. c. All choices may be found in patients with instability. However, a positive apprehension sign is the most sensitive for even subtle instability. Pain without apprehension in abduction, external rotation, and extension is indicative of impingement rather than instability.

35-6. c. Acromioclavicular separations can sometimes be tolerated for a day or so by some athletes but not the others. The mechanism is quite characteristic and in itself would implicate the acromioclavicular joint.

35-7. a. The mechanism of injury, position of joint stress, and the instant dysfunction tells you this must be an anterior dislocation. This can be seen in persons with very strong shoulders; one implication is that the pectoralis muscles can lever the humeral head anteriorly out of the glenoid cavity when the arm is in the vulnerable position.

35-8. d. The coracoid process can be injured with direct blows.

CHAPTER 36

Brachial Plexus Injuries

Robert E. Sallis, MD

QUESTIONS

36-1. With regard to transient brachial plexopathies, which of the following are true?
   a. commonly referred to as stingers.
   b. over 50% of football players may suffer this injury during their career.
   c. may be caused by a stretch of the brachial plexus.
   d. may be caused by a pinch of the brachial plexus.
   e. all of the above.

36-2. The symptoms of transient brachial plexopathy include:
   a. sudden burning pain and numbness down the lateral arm, thumb, and index finger.
   b. burning pain down both arms.
   c. severe weakness of one arm without pain.
   d. pain and numbness in the first three digits of the hand.
   e. pain which is worsened by lifting the arm above the head.

36-3. Football players with recurrent transient brachial plexopathy:
   a. should not be allowed to play.
   b. should be started on a rehabilitation program of the neck and shoulder.

c. should be encouraged to hit with the top of their helmet.

d. should wear smaller shoulder pads.

e. b and d.

36-4. Common sites for compression of the neurovascular bundle in the thoracic outlet include all, EXCEPT:

a. between the anterior and middle scalene muscles.

b. between the first rib and acromion.

c. under a cervical rib.

d. under the acromial arch.

e. all of the above are sites of compression.

36-5. Acute brachial neuropathy (or brachial plexitis):

a. is caused by an idiopathic inflammation of the brachial plexus.

b. is associated with intense shoulder pain and paresthesias.

c. is diagnosed by abnormal electromyogram.

d. is best treated conservatively.

e. all of the above.

ANSWERS

36-1. e. Transient brachial plexopathies (also known as stingers or burners) are a very common sports injury, especially in football, where up to 65% of players have them during their career. They are generally caused by forced lateral flexion of the head that results in either a stretch or a pinch of the brachial plexus.

36-2. a. Symptoms of transient brachial plexopathy include a sudden burning pain and numbness along the lateral arm, thumb, and index finger. This is accompanied by weakness of the deltoid, biceps, supraspinatus, and infraspinatus. These symptoms typically resolve after 1 or 2 minutes. Bilateral symptoms are indicative of transient quadriplegia (often associated with spinal stenosis).

36-3. b. Players with recurrent transient brachial plexopathy may return to play if all symptoms have resolved. They should be started on a rehabilitation program to strengthen neck and shoulder muscles. Hitting with the top of the helmet (spearing) is often a cause of this injury and is to be avoided. Larger shoulder pads that fit just under the helmet may help prevent this injury by decreasing lateral bending of the neck.

36-4. d. The subacromial space is not in the area of the thoracic outlet. Compression occurring here is on the rotator cuff tendons and causes the impingement syndrome. The other sites listed are all common sites of neurovascular compression in the thoracic outlet syndrome.

36-5. e. Brachial plexitis is an idiopathic inflammation of the brachial plexus characterized by intense shoulder pain and paresthesias, along with weakness of the proximal shoulder muscles. The electromyogram is abnormal, while laboratory tests (such as ESR and complete blood count) are normal. Most affected individuals improve with conservative treatment over weeks to years.

CHAPTER **37**

Rehabilitation of Shoulder Injuries

David B. Richards, MD

W. Benjamin Kibler, MD

QUESTIONS

37-1. Which of the following is true concerning shoulder stability?
   a. the anatomy of the shoulder makes it inherently stable.
   b. because the shoulder actually generates very little muscular force, stability is of minor importance.
   c. both static and dynamic constraints act continuously to maintain shoulder stability throughout a variety of activities.
   d. the unstable shoulder is easily recognized because of its recurrent dislocations.

37-2. Which of the following is true concerning shoulder rehabilitation?
   a. strength should be the top priority.
   b. normal shoulder function should be achieved before returning to competition.
   c. full range of motion (ROM) is the greatest concern.
   d. as soon as the patient is pain free, rehabilitation may be discontinued.

37-3. The most important element(s) of the shoulder rehabilitation program is (are):
   a. strength-building exercises.
   b. flexibility training.

c. neuromuscular training.

d. all of the above.

37-4. Once an acute anterior glenohumeral dislocation is reduced, the next phase of rehabilitation is:

a. rest, ice, elevation, compression.

b. prolonged rest to allow tissue healing.

c. gentle near-full ROM exercises, with light resistance.

d. aggressive strength training.

e. steroid injections.

ANSWERS

37-1. c. The shoulder is inherently unstable due to the large humeral head and shallow glenoid. The static constraints (labrum, capsule, and glenoid) and dynamic constraints (rotator cuff and scapula stabilizing muscles) act continuously in an attempt to maintain the center of rotation of the humeral head in the center of the glenoid. Chronic overload injuries to these constraints can lead to subtle instability with secondary impingement and damage to the labrum, without a frank dislocation. The shoulder funnels tremendous force from the legs and trunk out to the hand and has a very large range of motion. For this reason, shoulder stability is extremely important, especially in overhead sports.

37-2. b. Normal shoulder function is the goal of the rehabilitation program. This includes pain-free ROM, full strength and successful completion of sport-specific drills that develop muscle balance and firing patterns, and proprioception.

37-3. d. Shoulder rehabilitation is a complex process that requires a variety of methods to achieve optimum outcome. Strengthening exercises, both open and closed chain, are essential to normal shoulder function. The shoulder has the greatest active ROM of any joint in the body, and this should be maintained throughout the rehabilitation process. Normal muscle firing patterns around the shoulder are complex. Only through intensive neuromuscular training can these patterns be reestablished after injury.

37-4. c. Try applying ice, elevation, and compression to the shoulder; it is not easy. Do not keep the shoulder elevated. Prolonged rest does not promote tissue healing anywhere; active tissues heal better. Near full ROM is recommended to reduce the problems of contracture and keeps the joint healthy through surface contacts. Gentle strength training, even early, is recommended but aggressive training is not. Steroid injections are not used in acute injuries.

CHAPTER **38**

Anatomy and Biomechanics of the Elbow and Forearm

Michael D. Jackson, MD

Douglas B. McKeag, MD

QUESTIONS

38-1. Forearm pronation and supination are made possible primarily by movement of which articulations:
   a. humeroulnar and humeroradial joints.
   b. humeroulnar and inferior radioulnar joints.
   c. humeroulnar and superior radioulnar joints.
   d. humeroradial and inferior radioulnar joints.
   e. superior and inferior radioulnar joints.

38-2. Valgus instability of the elbow results when there is compromise of which ligament:
   a. lateral ulnar collateral ligament.
   b. posterior bundle of the medial ulnar collateral ligament.
   c. transverse bundle of the medial ulnar collateral ligament.
   d. anterior bundle of the medial ulnar collateral ligament.
   e. annular ligament.

38-3. Elbow flexion and forearm supination may be accomplished by which muscle:
   a. brachialis.
   b. biceps brachii.
   c. supinator.
   d. brachioradialis.

38-4. An athlete who complains of inability to flex the index and middle fingers, weakness on forearm pronation, wrist flexion, and numbness in the thumb, index, middle, and ring fingers may have injured which of the following nerves:
   a. musculocutaneous.
   b. ulnar.
   c. median.
   d. radial.

38-5. Flexion of the elbow ranges for 0 (full extension) to approximately 150 degrees of flexion, but this flexion range may be reduced by:
   a. tension of the elbow flexors.
   b. tension of the forearm pronator muscles.
   c. muscle mass of the anterior arm.
   d. tension of the interosseous membrane.

38-6. The muscle most commonly incriminated in lateral epicondylitis (tennis elbow) is:
   a. brachioradialis.
   b. middle extensor digitorum longus.
   c. extensor carpi radialis longus.
   d. extensor carpi radialis brevis.

ANSWERS

38-1. e. The superior and inferior radioulnar joints' primary action is to allow pronation and supination of the forearm. The humeroulnar joint's primary action is flexion and extension of the elbow. The humeroradial joint's primary action is also flexion and extension of the elbow, but it also acts in association with the superior radioulnar joint to allow the rotation necessary for pronation and supination.

38-2. d. Compromise of the anterior bundle of the medial ulnar collateral ligament results in valgus instability of the elbow in all positions except full extension. The lateral ulnar collateral ligament prevents inferior rotatory subluxation of the humeroulnar joint. The posterior bundle of the medial ulnar collateral ligament contributes to valgus instability when the elbow is flexed greater than 90 degrees. The transverse bundle of the medial ulnar collateral ligament plays no role in elbow stability. The annular ligament stabilizes the radial head in the radial notch of the ulna.

38-3. b. While primarily an elbow flexor, the biceps brachii also aids in supination. The brachialis and brachioradialis muscles are purely elbow flexors. The supinator muscle is purely a supinator.

38-4. c. The median nerve innervates the finger flexors (flexor digitorum superficialis and flexor digitorum profundus of the index and ring finger), the forearm pronators (pronator teres and pronator quadratus), and one wrist flexor (flexor carpi radialis), while providing sensation to the thumb, index, middle, and half of the ring finger. The musculocutaneous nerve innervates the biceps brachii, brachialis, and coracobrachialis, while providing sensation to the anterolateral forearm. The ulnar nerve innervates one wrist flexor (flexor carpi ulnaris), finger flexors on the ring and fifth finger, and the majority of hand intrinsic muscles, while providing sensation in half the ring and the entire fifth finger. The radial nerve innervates the wrist extensors and provides sensation on the dorsum of the hand.

38-5. c. Elbow flexion can be limited by muscle mass of the anterior arm and contact of the coronoid process with the coronoid fossa. Tension of the elbow flexors limits the range of elbow extension. Tension of the forearm pronator muscles may limit forearm supination. Tension of the interosseous membrane may limit both pronation and supination of the forearm.

38-6. d. The extensor carpi radialis brevis attaches directly onto the lateral epicondyle through an aponeurosis-like tendon. The weakest link in the chain is at the enthes, just 1 mm or so distal to the bone-tendon junction. This is the location of the microtears that are associated with avulsion strains through the extensor carpi radialis brevis. Other muscles can play a role as well, sometimes the long extensor digitorum muscles.

CHAPTER **39**

History and Physical Examination of the Elbow and Forearm

Michael D. Jackson, MD

Douglas B. McKeag, MD

QUESTIONS

39-1. When visually inspecting the elbow, the carrying angle should be noted; this normally measures:
   a. approximately 5 degrees in females.
   b. 10-15 degrees in males.
   c. greater than 10 degrees in males.
   d. less than 10 degrees in females.
   e. approximately 5 degrees in males.

39-2. When testing forearm flexion, which of the following positions best allows for testing of the biceps brachii?
   a. forearm supinated.
   b. forearm pronated.
   c. forearm in the midposition.
   d. forearm pronated and the wrist flexed.

39-3. The C6 nerve root can be evaluated by testing the:
   a. biceps reflex.
   b. brachioradialis reflex.
   c. triceps reflex.
   d. patellar reflex.
   e. ankle jerk reflex.

39-4. Provocative tests for lateral epicondylitis include:
   a. varus stress.
   b. resistance to wrist flexion.
   c. resistance to extension of the second digit.
   d. extension of the elbow with the wrist palmar flexed and the forearm fully pronated.
   e. extension of the elbow with the wrist dorsiflexed and the forearm fully supinated.

39-5. Ligamentous stability of the elbow is best evaluated with the elbow in:
   a. greater than 90 degrees of flexion.
   b. full extension.
   c. approximately 10 degrees of flexion.
   d. approximately 20 degrees of flexion.
   e. approximately 30 degrees of flexion.

ANSWERS

39-1. e. The carrying angle is the valgus angle formed by the longitudinal axes of the upper arm and forearm when the arm is fully extended in the anatomical position. In females the normal angle is 10-15 degrees, while in males the normal angle is approximately 5 degrees.

39-2. a. The biceps brachii is specifically tested while the patient flexes the elbow with the forearm supinated. Elbow flexion against resistance with the forearm pronated tests the brachialis muscle. With the forearm in the midposition, elbow flexion against resistance tests the brachioradialis. Adding wrist flexion does not help differentiate between the primary elbow flexors.

39-3. b. The brachioradialis reflex, which is elicited at the brachioradialis tendon at the distal end of the radius, evaluates the C6 nerve root. The biceps reflex, elicited at the biceps tendon in the cubital fossa, evaluates the C5 nerve root. The triceps reflex, elicited where the triceps tendon crosses the olecranon fossa, evaluates the C7 nerve root.

39-4. d. Provocative tests for lateral epicondylitis include tests that stress muscles of the common extensor group that originates from the lateral epicondyle, especially the extensor carpi radialis brevis. These tests include resistance to wrist extension, resistance to extension of the third digit, and extension of the elbow with the wrist palmar flexed and the forearm fully pronated. Varus stress of the elbow tests lateral ligament complex stability. Resistance to wrist flexion stresses the common flexor group that originates from the medial epicondyle. Resistance to extension of the second digit stresses the extensor indices that originate from the body of the ulna. Extension of the elbow with the wrist dorsiflexed and the forearm fully supinated also tests the common flexor group as they originate from the medial epicondyle.

39-5. e. Ligamentous stability of the elbow is evaluated with varus and valgus stress at approximately 30 degrees of flexion, as this unlocks the olecranon tip from the olecranon fossa. With the elbow flexed at ≥90 degrees the posterior bundle of the medial collateral ligament complex becomes taut, thus making it difficult to detect laxity in the primary stabilizers. From full extension to approximately 30 degrees of flexion the olecranon tip is positioned in the olecranon fossa, therefore making it more difficult to elicit ligamentous laxity.

CHAPTER 40

Injuries About the Elbow

Walter L. Calmbach, MD

Jorge Gomez, MD

QUESTIONS

40-1. The muscle that is primarily involved in lateral epicondylitis is the:
   a. extensor carpi radialis longus.
   b. extensor carpi radialis brevis.
   c. extensor digitorum communis.
   d. extensor carpi ulnaris.
   e. biceps brachii.

40-2. Osteochondritis dissecans most commonly affects the:
   a. proximal ulna.
   b. distal ulna.
   c. radiocapitellar joint.
   d. humeral trochlea.
   e. medial epicondyle.

40-3. The likelihood of developing myositis ossificans after elbow dislocation is increased by:
   a. prompt, gentle reduction.
   b. immobilization for 10-21 days.
   c. early active range of motion (ROM) exercises.
   d. early passive ROM exercises.
   e. intact neurovascular function.

40-4. A nondisplaced radial head fracture should be treated with:
  a. aspirate hemarthrosis, brief immobilization, early ROM.
  b. aspirate hemarthrosis, splint elbow for 21 days.
  c. steroid injection to relieve swelling.
  d. arthroscopic removal of bony fragments.
  e. open reduction, internal fixation.

40-5. A posterior elbow dislocation most commonly injures:
  a. the radial nerve and radial artery.
  b. the radial nerve and brachial artery.
  c. the median nerve and brachial artery.
  d. the median nerve and radial artery.
  e. the ulnar nerve and brachial artery.

ANSWERS

40-1. b. While all the muscles of the extensor-supinator mass may be involved to some degree, the extensor carpi radialis brevis (ECRB) is the primary cause of the symptoms of lateral epicondylitis. Of the two extensors that also abduct the wrist (the ECRB and the extensor carpi radialis longus [ECRL]) only the ECRB originates from the common extensor tendon at the lateral epicondyle (the ECRL originates from the lateral margin of the humerus proximal to the epicondyle).

40-2. c. Osteochondritis dissecans most commonly affects the radio-capitellar joint due to the tremendous valgus stresses placed on the elbow during the cocking and acceleration phases of throwing. This causes repeated compression at the lateral aspect of the elbow joint, predisposing the athlete to osteochondritis dissecans.

40-3. d. Myositis ossificans is a serious complication of some cases of elbow dislocation and can be worsened by passive ROM exercises because this may stimulate osteogenic elements displaced into the soft tissues during dislocation. Active ROM exercises are safer because pain limits ROM during the early phase of healing.

40-4. a. A nondisplaced radial head fracture should be treated by aspirating the hemarthrosis, because this alleviates pain and allows early ROM. Brief immobilization in a sling for <3 days is usually sufficient, and prolonged immobilization can lead to joint stiffness and decreased ROM. Early ROM exercises are indicated because loss of full extension (~10 degrees) is a common complication of this injury.

40-5. c. Posterior elbow dislocation can cause injury to the median nerve and brachial artery. The median nerve can be stretched or may become caught between displaced bony elements. The brachial artery may be torn or, more commonly, the dislocation causes injury and spasm at the brachial artery. If unrecognized and untreated, this may lead to the disabling Volkmann's ischemic contracture.

CHAPTER **41**

History and Physical Exam
Murray E. Allen, MD

QUESTIONS

41-1. Weakness of opposing thumb and fifth finger is an indicator of involvement of which nerve:
a. radial.
b. median.
c. ulnar.

41-2. Weakness of finger abduction is an indicator of involvement of which nerve:
a. radial.
b. median.
c. ulnar.

41-3. Numbness of the index and middle finger may be an indicator of:
a. carpal tunnel syndrome.
b. thoracic outlet syndrome.
c. Guyon's canal entrapment neuropathy.
d. de Quervain's disorder.
e. repetitive strain disorder.

41-4. The most common scaphoid fracture involves the:
a. distal one third.

       b. midbelly.

       c. proximal one third.

41-5. The slowest healing of scaphoid fractures involves the:
       a. distal one third.
       b. midbelly.
       c. proximal one third.

41-6. The key time for confirmatory radiographic diagnosis of a sus-pected scaphoid fracture is:
       a. at the time of injury, day 1.
       b. day 5.
       c. day 10.
       d. 3 months.
       e. 6 months.

41-7. "Intersection" syndrome is:
       a. de Quervain's tenosynovitis of the dorsal radial wrist.
       b. carpal tunnel syndrome of the volar carpal tunnel.
       c. midbelly scaphoid injury of the radial wrist.
       d. adductor injury to the ulnar thumb ligament.
       e. tenosynovitis between the first and second dorsal wrist compartment.

41-8. The diagnosis of carpal tunnel syndrome is confirmed by:
       a. Tinel's sign.
       b. Phalen's test.
       c. history of repetitive strain causing wrist and hand pain.
       d. nerve conduction delay.
       e. numb fingers with wrist pain.

41-9. Injury to the distal neck of the fifth metacarpal:
       a. always requires pinning to return the metacarpal to perfect alignment, which is quite necessary.
       b. can usually be reduced to reasonable adequacy by fixing with the joint flexed.

41-10. "Mallet" finger is:
       a. an avulsion of the fingernail.
       b. a crush-type injury to the fingernail with subungual hematoma.
       c. a third degree tear of the dorsal hood of the middle interpha-langeal (MIP) joint.
       d. an avulsion of the dorsal tendon from the distal phalanx.
       e. flexor digital tendinitis seen in carpenters.

41-11. A tear of the ulnar collateral ligament of the metacarpophalangeal (MCP) joint of the thumb can be a:
       a. gamekeeper's thumb.
       b. skier's thumb.
       c. Stener lesion.
       d. surgical condition.
       e. all of the above.

ANSWERS

41-1. b. The median nerve subserves the thenar eminence, a powerful opposer.

41-2. c. The ulnar nerve also subserves adduction, but abduction is easier to test and compare side to side.

41-3. a. True carpal tunnel syndrome is an entrapment neuropathy of the median nerve, which causes numbness to index and middle fingers. Confirming this diagnosis requires nerve studies, showing conduction delay across the carpal tunnel. Other noncarpal tunnel–type pain can be confused with carpal tunnel but will lack the nerve conduction delay.

41-4. b. The midbelly of the scaphoid is fractured most frequently, about 70%. The distal scaphoid is fractured about 10%, and the proximal about 20%.

41-5. c. The blood supply to the scaphoid comes from the distal portion; the proximal is the least supplied and the slowest to heal, at least up to 16 weeks. Proximal scaphoid fractures should be cast, including the thumb and elbow with a long arm cast, at least for the first month.

41-6. c. The suspected scaphoid fracture should be treated with cast immobilization including the thumb, until proven otherwise. At 10 days, radiography will show a positive fracture line or, conversely, exclude the diagnosis.

41-7. e. Intersection syndrome is a dorsal compartment tenosynovitis, sometimes with quite loud crepitus that is sometimes called "squeaker's wrist." It is a repetitive strain disorder.

41-8. d. The diagnosis of carpal tunnel syndrome requires a significant delay across the carpal tunnel; all other signs and symptoms can also occur with various other noncarpal tunnel aches and pains.

41-9. b. Boxer's fractures of the distal fifth metacarpal neck usually reduce when the joint is flexed and then fixed at this position. Flexion angulation up to 70 degrees can sometimes be tolerated.

41-10. d. The mallet finger gets its name from the characteristic shape of the distal interphalangeal joint (DIP) after a flexion strain at that joint, which avulses the dorsal tendon attachment, with or without bone. Surgery is often an option but is not always successful in reducing the mallet deformity.

41-11. e. Skier's or gamekeeper's thumb is often a surgical disorder due to interposition of the adductor aponeurosis between the torn ligament ends; this is known as a Stener lesion. Both early or late surgery is effective in restoring functional stability to this important joint.

Wrist and Hand Injuries in Sports

Robert J. Dimeff, MD

QUESTIONS

42-1. A player falls backward onto his outstretched hands. He complains of pain in both wrists but is able to continue participation. After the game he notices swelling and pain at the dorsal radial aspect of the wrist. Examination reveals a loss of wrist and thumb extension and swelling and tenderness between the abductor pollicis longus (APL)/extensor pollicis brevis (EPB) tendons and the extensor pollicis longus (EPL) tendon. Initial radiographs are normal. The most likely diagnosis is:
   a. radioscapholunate dissociation.
   b. stenosing tenosynovitis.
   c. scaphoid fracture.
   d. hook of the hamate fracture.
   e. triangular fibrocartilage complex tear.

42-2. Scapholunate dissociation is the most common significant wrist sprain. All of the following are true regarding this injury, EXCEPT:
   a. the mechanism of injury is a fall on the outstretched hand.
   b. clenched fist PA radiographs will reveal 3 mm or more separation between the scaphoid and lunate bones.
   c. it may occur as a result of a tear of the volar radioscapholunate ligament or as a result of nonunion of a scaphoid fracture.

    d. radioscapholunate angle <30 degrees.

    e. the treatment of choice of acute injuries is surgical repair.

42-3. Intersection syndrome:
    a. is due to repetitive axial loading of the extended wrist.
    b. is due to irritation of the extensor pollicis longus tendon as it passes around Lister's tubercle on the dorsal aspect of the distal radius.
    c. is stenosing tenosynovitis of the APL and EPB tendons in the first dorsal compartment of the wrist.
    d. refers to an inflammatory condition at the junction of the muscles and tendons of the first and second dorsal compartment.
    e. results in isolated thumb–index finger pinch weakness without sensory changes.

42-4. An 18-year-old gymnast complains of a 3-month history of increasing dorsoulnar wrist pain with occasional swelling. Her symptoms are exacerbated with repeated wrist extension. She denies specific trauma. Her examination reveals a loss of 5 degrees of wrist extension with exquisite tenderness between the distal radius and ulna. Pain is also reproduced with passive wrist extension and ulnar deviation. No clicking is noted about the wrist. Wrist radiographs reveal no bone abnormalities. The ulna is 1 mm longer than the radius. Following a period of relative rest, immobilization, antiinflammatory medications, and cryotherapy the patient is able to return to participation. However, she develops recurrence of her symptoms. You recommend the following treatment based on an MRI scan that confirms your suspected diagnosis:
    a. cortisone injection into the fourth dorsal compartment.
    b. debridement of the triangular fibrocartilage complex with concomitant distal ulnar resection.
    c. open reduction internal fixation with bone graft.
    d. triscaphe (scapho-trapezial-trapezoid) effusion.
    e. none of the above.

42-5. All of the following are true regarding carpal fractures, EXCEPT:
    a. hook of the hamate fractures may require surgical intervention.
    b. pisiform fractures are prone to nonunion.
    c. avascular necrosis is a complication of lunate fracture.
    d. scaphoid fractures occur most commonly in the distal third.
    e. none of the above.

42-6. A basketball player presents with a history of jamming his middle finger with a basketball. He is complaining of pain and swelling of the proximal interphalangeal (PIP) joint of the middle finger. The examination reveals loss of 20 degrees of extension, swelling of the PIP joint and diffuse tenderness, dorsal greater than volar. There is no crepitus, angulation, or rotational deformity. The most likely diagnosis is:
    a. nondisplaced fracture of the middle phalanx.

b. extensor mechanism injury.

c. dorsal dislocation of the PIP with spontaneous reduction.

d. volar plate avulsion fracture.

e. pseudo-boutonniére deformity.

42-7. A snow skier falls forward onto his outstretched hand; the ski pole forces his thumb into abduction. He presents with complaints of pain and swelling of the right thumb and hand. All of the following statements are true regarding this injury, EXCEPT:

    a. ligament stability is best tested with the metacarpophalangeal (MCP) joint flexed.

    b. radiography should be performed prior to ligament stress testing.

    c. the adductor pollicis aponeurosis may interpose between the torn ends of the ulnar collateral ligament (UCL).

    d. nondisplaced avulsion fractures should be treated with thumb spica immobilization.

    e. surgery should be performed on second degree sprains to decrease recovery time.

42-8. A blow to the tip of the finger such as getting the finger jammed with a softball may produce a mallet deformity. All of the following are true, EXCEPT:

    a. this injury involves the extensor mechanism to the distal interphalangeal (DIP) joint.

    b. the patient has full passive range of motion of the PIP and DIP joints.

    c. the finger should be splinted in 30 degrees of flexion for 4-6 weeks.

    d. the athlete will have point tenderness over the dorsum of the DIP.

42-9. All of the following are true regarding metacarpal fractures, EXCEPT:

    a. fracture of the base of the thumb due to adduction stress may lead to subluxation of the trapezium-thumb metacarpal joint requiring surgical stabilization.

    b. rotational malalignment is best observed with the MCP fully extended.

    c. 40 degrees of dorsal angulation is acceptable with fifth metacarpal shaft fractures.

    d. metacarpal shaft fractures associated with 4 mm of shortening require surgical stabilization.

42-10. All of the following are true, EXCEPT:

    a. ulnar nerve compression in cyclists may cause either motor or sensory abnormalities in the fourth and fifth digits.

    b. hypertrophy of the flexor digitorum superficialis may lead to compression of the median nerve, causing hand pain and dysesthesia of the first, second, and third digits.

c. weakness of wrist and MCP extension may be due to posterior interosseous nerve entrapment.

d. superficial radial nerve compression (Wartenberg's disease = cheiralgia paresthetica) results in dysesthesia of the dorsal radial aspect of the hand and index finger with weakness of thumb extension.

42-11. In an athlete who presents with history of trauma to the PIP joint of the index finger with tenderness over the dorsal aspect of the joint, you should consider the possibility of:

a. a dislocation of the PIP joint with spontaneous reduction.
b. a volar plate fracture.
c. an injury to the dorsal hood.
d. acute traumatic capsulitis of the PIP joint.
e. undisplaced fracture of the middle phalanx.

42-12. A fall on the outstretched hand, which causes tenderness deep between the abductor pollicis longus–extensor pollicis brevis tendons and the extensor pollicis longus tendon, could be an indication of:

a. ulnar nerve entrapment.
b. carpal tunnel syndrome.
c. fracture of scaphoid bone.
d. subluxation of lunate bone.
e. midwrist ligament sprain.

42-13. Management of the above possible disorder consists of:

a. radiography to exclude bony injury, surgical release of entrapping ligament.
b. radiography to confirm, wrist cast even if negative, and repeat x-ray in 2 weeks.
c. radiography to confirm, open surgical reduction.
d. radiography to exclude other injury, wrist splint for comfort.

42-14. Placing the back of the hands together with slight pressure, then pushing the wrists together in forced passive flexion, pointing the fingers towards the chest in a position known as the Phalen's test, causes compression of the:

a. ulnar nerve.
b. median nerve.
c. radial nerve.

42-15. In Phalen's test, you are checking for:

a. tennis elbow.
b. Reynaud's syndrome.
c. cervical radiculopathy.
d. carpal tunnel syndrome.
e. Colles' fracture.

42-16. Guyon's canal at the volar wrist carries a branch of the ulnar nerve. A neuropathy here with a positive Tinel's sign is often seen in which athletes?

a. elite level carpet bowlers on the down hand.
b. cyclists, both or either hand.
c. tennis players, playing hand.
d. archers, on the push forward hand.

ANSWERS

42-1. c. Scaphoid fracture. The scaphoid bone articulates with the distal radius, lunate, capitate, trapezium, and trapezoid. Because of its anatomical position this bone is prone to fracture when an axial load is applied across the extended wrist. The most common clinical findings are swelling and tenderness of the anatomical snuffbox. Seventy percent of the fractures are through the middle third or waist, 20% are proximal, and 10% are distal. Proximal fractures are prone to avascular necrosis. The initial radiographs are usually normal. Bone scan or computerized tomography (CT) or magnetic resonance imaging (MRI) scan may assist in confirming a diagnosis. Alternatively, the patient may be treated with thumb spica immobilization for 10-14 days followed by repeat radiography. Confirmed nondisplaced fractures should be treated with thumb spica immobilization, initially a long arm cast for 2 weeks, followed by a short arm cast for 6-8 weeks, until the fracture is clinically and radiographically healed. Alternatively, nondisplaced midwaist fractures may be treated with internal fixation with compressive screw with early return to participation.

Scapholunate dissociation results from an injury to the palmar radioscapholunate ligament or a chronic scaphoid nonunion. This injury may also occur acutely from a fall on the outstretched hand; however, the area of tenderness is at a more ulnar location, not specific to the snuffbox, and radiography reveals widening >3 mm between the scaphoid and lunate bones. Stenosing tenosynovitis of the APL and EPB tendons of the first dorsal compartment of the wrist (also known as de Quervain's disease) is due to repeated forceful gripping with radial and ulnar deviation or repetitive thumb activity. Finkelstein's test, in which the thumb is flexed into the palm while the examiner ulnarly deviates the wrist, will reproduce symptoms. Hook of the hamate fractures are due to direct trauma to the hypothenar aspect of the hand, usually from a racquet or baseball bat. Swelling and tenderness are localized to the hypothenar aspect of the hand. Triangular fibrocartilage complex tears result from repeated hyperpronation of the forearm with axial load of the wrist. This injury may occur as an acute traumatic event or from chronic repeated stress. Symptoms include dorsal ulnar wrist pain exacerbated with wrist extension and ulnar deviation and tenderness localized to the region of the distal radial ulnar joint (DRUJ). Radiography often reveals positive ulnar variance.

42-2. d. Scapholunate dissociation is most commonly the result of a fall on an outstretched hand. The athlete will present with a loss of wrist extension, swelling, and tenderness in the region of the radioscapholunate articulation. Comparison films, including stress films, are often necessary to confirm the diagnosis. Clenched fist PA radiography will reveal >3 mm separation between the scaphoid and lunate bone or a space two times that of other carpal spaces. The normal radioscapholunate angle is 30 to 60 degrees. An angle <30 degrees is referred to as palmar intercalated segment instability (PISI), and an angle >70 degrees refers to dorsiflexed intercalated segment instability (DISI). A tear of the ligaments between the scaphoid and the lunate will allow the lunate to extend (dorsiflex) away from its normal articulation with the scaphoid; hence there is an increase in the radioscapholunate angle. Acute scapholunate dissociation should be treated with soft tissue repair and possible K-wire flexion. Chronic instability due to unrecognized dissociation or nonunion of a scaphoid fracture usually requires fusion of the scaphoid to the trapezium and trapezoid bones (triscaphe fusion).

42-3. d. Intersection syndrome is described as an inflammatory condition located at the crossing points between the first dorsal compartment (APL and EPB) and the second dorsal compartment (extensor carpi radialis longus [ECRL] and extensor carpi radialis brevis [ECRB]) muscles. This condition is characterized by pain and swelling approximately 4-6 cm proximal to the radiocarpal joint, often associated with palpable audible crepitus, hence the name "squeakers." It most commonly affects oarsmen and those involved in weight training with repetitive wrist flexion/extension and thumb extensions. Four different pathophysiological theories have been proposed: (1) acute inflammation of the APL and EPB muscle bellies; (2) friction leading to the development of inflamed adventitial bursa between the APL and the ECRB, (3) tenosynovitis of the ECRL and the ECRB; and (4) exertional compartment syndrome of the APL and the EPB. Standard treatment includes relative rest, ice, nonsteroidal antiinflammatory drugs, rehabilitation exercises, thumb spica immobilization including night splints, cortisone injection, and possible surgical exploration if symptoms do not resolve.

Intersection syndrome is caused by repeated wrist extension rather than axial load. EPL tendinitis is due to friction that develops as the tendon passes around Lister's tubercle; because this tendon is prone to rupture, cortisone should not be administered. Surgical treatment for chronic cases involves transposing the EPL to the opposite side of Lister's tubercle. Stenosing tenosynovitis of the first dorsal compartment (APL and EPB tendons) is de Quervain's syndrome. Inflammatory changes are localized to the first dorsal compartment of the wrist, and Finkelstein's test is positive. Treatment is similar to that for intersection syndrome. Weakness of thumb-finger pinch is related to anterior interosseous nerve entrapment, leading to weakness of the flexor digitorum profundus of the second digit, flexor pollicis longus (FPL), and pronator quadratus with no sensory deficits.

42-4. b. Triangular fibrocartilage complex (TFCC) tears may occur as a result of a traumatic injury or chronic repetition. Hyperpronation of the forearm in conjunction with axial load increases the stress across the wrist joint. Complaints include pain and tenderness at the DRUJ that are worse at the extremes of forearm pronation and supination, with radial/ulnar compression, and with dorsal/volar translation of the ulna. The radius normally transmits approximately 80% of the axial load across the wrist and the ulna 20%. If the ulna is increased 2.5 mm in length, 60% of the load is transferred through the radius and 40% through the ulna. Positive ulnar variance refers to the fact that the ulna is longer than the radius. Patients with TFCC tears will usually have a normal radiograph; however, PA views may reveal positive ulnar variance. Arthrogram and MRI scan can confirm the diagnosis. If conservative management fails to improve symptoms, recommended surgical treatment includes debridement of the TFCC and possibly ulnar shortening.

Cortisone injection into the fourth dorsal compartment may be helpful for extensor digitorum communis and extensor indices tendinitis. Open reduction internal fixation with bone grafting would most likely be performed in cases of nonunion of the scaphoid fracture. Triscaphe fusion is the most common wrist arthrodesis and is usually performed to treat chronic wrist instability secondary to scaphoid nonunion or scapholunate dissociation.

42-5. d. Hook of the hamate fractures are due to a direct blow to the hyperthenar region of the hand or from the impact of a racquet or bat. Examination will reveal localized swelling and tenderness. Carpal tunnel or supination oblique radiography may be necessary to reveal the fracture. Occasionally, bone scan and CT are required for the diagnosis. Excision of the fracture is the preferred treatment in the athlete who is usually able to return to participation within 4-8 weeks.

Pisiform fractures are rare, may be due to direct trauma, and are prone to nonunion as the pisiform is a sesamoid bone within the flexor carpi ulnaris tendon. The injury may be treated with cast immobilization; however, surgical excision may be necessary. Lunate fractures, like proximal pole of the scaphoid fractures, are prone to avascular necrosis. These injuries must be monitored closely. Nondisplaced fractures are immobilized until radiographic evidence of healing occurs. Surgical intervention may be necessary for nonunion or avascular necrosis.

Seventy percent of scaphoid fractures are at the waist, 20% at the proximal pole, and 10% at the distal pole. Owing to the blood supply, the proximal scaphoid fractures are most prone to nonunion. Ninety-five percent or more of middle and distal scaphoid fractures will heal with proper treatment.

42-6. b. Rupture of the central slip of the extensor tendon over the PIP joint may lead to migration of the lateral bands volar to the axis of the joint. The mechanism is forced flexion of the actively extended PIP joint (jammed finger), direct trauma to the dorsum of the PIP, or previous volar PIP dislocation. The athlete will present with pain, swelling, tenderness of the PIP joint, loss of PIP motion, and extensor lag. Treatment requires 6-8 weeks of splinting with the PIP in full extension. Misdiagnosis may lead to a chronic boutonniére deformity in which there is a fixed flexion contracture of the PIP joint and fixed extension contracture of the DIP joint.

Nondisplaced fracture of the middle phalanx may present with hyperextension or axial loading mechanism; tenderness is localized to the area of the fracture rather than the joint. Dorsal dislocation of the PIP joint is the most common dislocation of the hand and is due to hyperextension causing disruption of the volar plate and tearing of the accessory collateral ligaments. Following reduction, the joint must be examined for collateral ligament stability. The joint should be splinted in slight flexion for 1-2 weeks. Hyperextension injuries may also be associated with an avulsion fracture of the volar plate. Isolated volar plate injuries are less common than those associated with full dislocation. The patient will present with a swollen PIP joint, decreased range of motion secondary to pain, and tenderness localized to the volar aspect of the middle phalanx. Radiography will confirm the diagnosis. Treatment is with the joint immobilized at 20-30 degrees of flexion for 2-3 weeks.

Pseudo-boutonniére deformity is a slowly progressive deformity of the PIP joint due to a previous volar plate injury. Calcification and scarring lead to a fixed flexion contracture of the PIP with slight unfixed hyperextension of the DIP. Treatment involves dynamic splinting; however, surgical release may be necessary for flexion contractures >40 degrees.

42-7. e. Thumb UCL sprain, also known as "skier's thumb," is the most common ligamentous injury to the thumb. The usual mechanism of injury is forced abduction of the thumb. The athlete will present with pain and swelling in the first web space, weakness of thumb index pinch, and tenderness along the UCL. A Stener lesion may be palpable just proximal to the MCP joint; this represents the adductor aponeurosis interpositioned between the torn ends of the UCL. Radiographs should be obtained prior to full stressing so as to decrease the risk of displacing a previously nondisplaced avulsion fracture; the avulsion fracture associated with UCL sprain is usually from the base of the proximal phalanx. Stress testing of the MCP joint should be performed at a variety of degrees of flexion; the UCL proper provides stability when the MP is flexed. A difference of 15 degrees of laxity compared to the contralateral side or >30 degrees of laxity is suggestive of a complete ligament tear (third-degree sprain). Treatment of first- and second-degree sprains requires thumb spica immobilization for 2-4 weeks with protection from abduction stress during activity. Nondisplaced avulsion fractures are treated with thumb spica immobilization for 4-6 weeks until the fracture heals. Avulsion fractures displaced >1 mm generally require surgical stabilization. Third-degree sprains without fracture may require surgical repair, either immediate or delayed; this is a controversial topic. Surgical intervention for partial UCL sprains has not been demonstrated to decrease recovery time.

42-8. c. Mallet finger is an injury to the extensor mechanism that occurs when an impact on the tip of the finger forces DIP flexion while the extensor mechanism is contracting. The extensor tendon may be stretched, ruptured, or associated with a small avulsion fracture, a large articular fracture, or a slipped epiphysis. The patient will present with localized swelling and tenderness of the DIP and dorsal aspect of the distal phalanx with inability to actively extend the DIP joint. This injury should be treated with the DIP in full extension for 6-8 weeks. Persistent volar subluxation of the distal phalanx or fractures involving >50% of the articular surface usually require surgical intervention. The athlete may return to participation with protective splinting.

42-9. b. Rotational alignment of metacarpal fractures is best tested with the MCP and IP fully flexed. Fracture at the base of metacarpal II through IV are usually stable due to the effects of intermetacarpal ligaments, intrinsic muscles, and fascia. However, a fracture at the base of the first metacarpal due to an adduction stress results in a Bennett's fracture. This is a fracture subluxation of the trapezium–first metacarpal joint and requires surgical fixation due to instability; the APL insertion at the base of the first metacarpal causes proximal displacement of the metacarpal shaft.

Stable metacarpal fractures may be treated with cast immobilization. Metacarpal fractures are considered stable if there is no rotatory malalignment, <3 mm of shortening, and satisfactory alignment (40-50 degrees of dorsal angulation is acceptable at metacarpal IV and V, no more than 15-20 degrees of dorsal angulation is acceptable at metacarpals II and III). Unstable fractures should be treated with surgical fixation and early motion. Alternatively, stable metacarpal fractures may be surgically stabilized to allow early motion and return to participation in those sports in which protective bracing is unacceptable.

42-10. d. The superficial radial nerve is a pure sensory nerve that supplies sensation to the dorsal aspect of the radial hand, thumb, and index finger. This is most commonly compressed by wearing tight wrist bands. This nerve has no motor branches. Guyon's canal syndrome or compression of the ulnar nerve in Guyon's canal is common in cyclists and presents with numbness and/or weakness of the ulnar one and a half digits. The pronator syndrome refers to compression of the median nerve in the proximal forearm that presents with proximal volar forearm ache, occasional hand pain, and dysesthesia of the radial three and a half digits supplied by the median nerve. The nerve may be compressed by the Struthers' ligament, the lacertus fibrosis, the pronator teres, or the proximal arch of the flexor digitorum superficialis. The posterior interosseous nerve pierces the forearm through the supinator. Entrapment of this distal branch of the radial nerve will cause vague lateral elbow and forearm pain, and may lead to weakness of wrist extension, MCP extension, and wrist ulnar deviation. This is a pure motor branch; as a result, there are no sensory deficits.

42-11. c. Dorsal hood injuries occur to the PIP joint. The dorsal hood is a complex structure with attachments to joint capsule as well as the extensor tendons, and remote attachments to the flexor tendons apparatus as well.

42-12. c. This is a repeat question on the all important scaphoid fracture, with tenderness deep in the anatomical muff bone.

42-13. b. Scaphoid fractures may not show up on the initial x-rays; therefore they must be repeated at the time when some fracture absorption will expose the defect. In the meantime the suspected scaphoid fracture should be cast. Since a fracture across the midbelly of the scaphoid can interrupt the blood supply to the proximal half, which gets its blood supply only from the distal half, excess motion across the fracture site could be disastrous and lead to aseptic necrosis of the proximal half. Long-term consequences of such an event are not good.

42-14. b. This is the classic test for compression in the carpal tunnel, which carries the median nerve.

42-15. d. However, mere presence of a positive Phalen's test does not confirm carpal tunnel syndrome, which must be diagnosed by electroconductive delays across the tunnel.

42-16. b. Tinel's sign merely means a short, sharp electric-type pain with radiations when tapping a nerve. Bash your funny bone (ulnar nerve to doctors) and you've self-imposed this sign. Cyclists often bruise a branch of the ulnar nerve at the volar wrist, and this can lead to an atrophy of intrinsic muscles of the hand, which at times has no sensory loss at all.

CHAPTER 43

Diagnosis and Management of Concussion

Robert C. Cantu, MD

QUESTIONS

43-1. Sports at greatest risk of head and spine injury include:
   a. football.
   b. ice hockey.
   c. gymnastics.
   d. all of the above.

43-2. With a mild concussion there is:
   a. no loss of consciousness and posttraumatic amnesia <30 minutes.
   b. no loss of consciousness and posttraumatic amnesia >30 minutes.
   c. no loss of consciousness and posttraumatic amnesia >24 hours.
   d. a brief loss of consciousness.

43-3. An athlete should not be allowed to return to a contact collision sport after a cerebral concussion if:
   a. <1 week has passed.
   b. the athlete has any postconcussion symptoms.
   c. <2 weeks have passed.
   d. there has been a prior concussion.

43-4. With a grade III concussion, an athlete may return to competition:
   a. after 1 month.

    b. after 1 month if asymptomatic for at least 1 week previously at rest and exertion.

    c. after 2 months.

    d. after 3 months.

43-5. With a grade II concussion, an athlete should be:

    a. removed from the contest but may return during the second half if asymptomatic.

    b. removed from the contest and allowed to sit on the bench but not return to the contest.

    c. removed from the contest and sent to the hospital for further neurological evaluation.

    d. evaluated with magnetic resonance imaging of the brain.

ANSWERS

43-1. d. Football, ice hockey and gymnastics are all among the sports at high risk of concussion.

43-2. a. With a mild or grade 1 concussion, there is no loss of consciousness, and posttraumatic amnesia, if present, is <30 minutes.

43-3. b. It is of the utmost importance that no athlete be allowed to return to contact collision sports if postconcussion symptoms are still present; to do so would put the athlete at risk of the second impact syndrome. It does not matter whether this requires 1 or 2 weeks or if there have been prior concussions. What is absolutely essential is that there be no postconcussion symptoms when the athlete is allowed to return to contact collision sports.

43-4. b. The crux is that the individual has been asymptomatic for at least 1 week at rest and exertion (a, c, and d make no mention of the need to be asymptomatic for 1 week at rest and exertion).

43-5. c. It is a clinical decision whether computerized tomography or magnetic resonance imaging of the head is necessary. Under no circumstances should the athlete be allowed to return to the contest, and the athlete should not remain on the bench.

CHAPTER 44

Field Management of Head Injuries and Return to Play

Roger L. McCoy II, MD

QUESTIONS

44-1. With any loss of consciousness, what associated injury must be assumed present in a head-injured athlete?
   a. nasal fracture.
   b. basilar skull fractures.
   c. chest wall injury.
   d. cervical spine injury.

44-2. An athlete at a football game sustains what you grade as a grade I concussion yet still has continued symptoms past 20 minutes; he previously sustained a grade I concussion 2 weeks ago. Two days later the athlete still has some slight headache upon visiting your office. Your next step in regard to this athlete should be:
   a. return to play immediately.
   b. retire from collision sports altogether.
   c. return to play 1 week from the above evaluation.
   d. return to play 1 week after all symptoms have completely resolved.

44-3. All of the following statements concerning the second impact syndrome are true, EXCEPT:
   a. the syndrome occurs in athletes in whom symptoms from the previous minor head injury have not resolved.

b. athletes usually suffer some form of postconcussional symptoms after the very first injury.

c. the second impact must be of greater force than the first impact.

d. the pathophysiology of second impact syndrome is thought to involve loss of autoregulation of the brain's blood supply, leading to vascular engorgement.

44-4. Which of the following would indicate a more severe head injury and possibly be related to the onset of postconcussion syndrome symptoms?

a. dizziness.

b. posttraumatic amnesia.

c. retrograde amnesia.

d. headache.

44-5. All of the following would be appropriate field tests to evaluate a recently head-injured athlete, EXCEPT:

a. orientation questions regarding person, place, and time of game and importance of game and team being played.

b. serial 7s or the ability to repeat digits in backwards order when given to them.

c. finger-to-nose coordination testing along with Romberg testing.

d. asking the patient who the 17th president of the United States was and what years he served.

ANSWERS

44-1. d. The forces necessary to cause unconsciousness in a patient or athlete are usually strong enough to also inflict damage on the cervical spine, depending on its position at the time of impact. With an unconscious athlete, the ability to fully ascertain neurological status is impaired and so the physician must assume the possibility of the worst outcome (in this case cervical spine injury and possible quadriplegia) and treat any unconsciousness with the assumption that a cervical spine injury could be present.

44-2. d. Based on the findings, it is appropriate not to return the athlete to play as his symptoms have continued 2 days after the concussion occurred. Guidelines from the Colorado Medical Society suggest not returning to play after a second grade I concussion for at least 1 week after being asymptomatic. Reasoning for most of the recommendations are to help prevent the catastrophic second impact syndrome.

44-3. e. With several reports in the literature concerning second impact syndrome, it has been found that a second blow may be remarkably minor and perhaps not even be directly related to the head yet cause just enough force to damage a brain that has not completely recovered from its first head injury. Swollen tissues are believed to be particularly fragile and prone to reinjury. Again, it is important to allow resolution of all postconcussive symptoms before allowing an athlete to return to play.

44-4. b. Retrograde amnesia is the inability to recall events prior to the injury as opposed to posttraumatic amnesia, which is the inability to recall events after the injury. Posttraumatic amnesia is usually associated with more severe concussions and can be a semipredictive sign of the chance that an athlete may have postconcussion syndrome following head injury.

44-5. d. Cerebellar testing along with orientation and memory testing is very appropriate in assessing athletes on the field; however, patients must be asked questions that are somewhat familiar to them and to yourself so that they may be able to have the opportunity to answer questions appropriately. Exertional testing should also be performed to see if any symptoms of head injury are reproduced prior to returning athletes to play. The 17th president question would probably be failed by 75% of normal doctors.

C H A P T E R **45**

Anatomy and Biomechanics

Evan S. Bass, MD

QUESTIONS

45-1. A football player receives a traumatic neck injury during a game. Tenderness is noted in the cervical spine posteriorly at the same approximate level of the Adam's apple (thyroid cartilage). On radiographs, the physician should be most suspicious of injury to the:
   a. third cervical vertebra.
   b. fourth cervical vertebra.
   c. fifth cervical vertebra.
   d. sixth cervical vertebra.

45-2. Following a diving accident into shallow water, tenderness bilaterally in the area between the angle of the mandible and the mastoid process indicates a possible:
   a. fracture of the posterior arch of the atlas (C1).
   b. fracture of the body of the atlas (C1).
   c. fracture of the transverse process of the axis (C2).
   d. fracture of the odontoid process of the axis (C2).

45-3. A 17-year-old football player suffers a hyperflexion injury to the neck. Symptoms and findings suggest a radiculopathy of the C7 and C8 nerve roots. Which of the following statements is false?
   a. the C7-C8 radiculopathy may produce numbness in the fingers.

b. a diminished triceps tendon test may be present.

c. radiography is needed to rule out a fracture of C8.

d. grip strength may also be affected.

45-4. The atlantoaxial joint accounts for approximately what percentage of the rotational range of motion of the neck?

a. 30%.

b. 50%.

c. 70%.

d. 90%.

45-5. The most effective tool at preventing cervical spine injuries in football is:

a. a thorough flexibility and strengthening program for the neck.

b. use of a neck roll.

c. use of a cowboy collar.

d. enforcing proper tackling technique.

45-6. A football player presents 1 week after a traumatic neck injury complaining of ongoing neck pain with motion. Lateral, anteroposterior, and open-mouth views completed on the day of injury were normal. Neurological examination is normal, and the only physical finding is lower cervical pain with motion. Your next best step is:

a. treat conservatively with antiinflammatory medication and range of motion exercises.

b. repeat the cervical spine series with oblique views.

c. obtain flexion and extension lateral radiographs of the neck, allowing the patient to initiate motion of his neck to its full limitations of motion.

d. obtain flexion and extension lateral radiographs of the neck with the cervical spine carefully manipulated and positioned by the physician or technician.

45-7. A teenager presents to the emergency room following a cliff diving accident into shallow water. He is slightly inebriated and tender behind the angle of the jaw and posterior occipital area. Lateral, anteroposterior, and open-mouth odontoid views of the neck are all normal. Neurological examination is normal. As the physician, your next best step is to:

a. order oblique view plain films of the neck.

b. obtain flexion and extension lateral radiographs of the neck, allowing the patient to initiate motion of his neck to its full limitations of motion.

c. obtain flexion and extension lateral radiographs of the neck with the cervical spine carefully manipulated and positioned by the physician or technician.

d. order a computerized tomography scan.

45-8. The most common mechanism of serious neck injury in football is:
   a. axial loading with neck slightly extended.
   b. axial loading with neck flexed forward slightly.
   c. hyperextension of the neck.
   d. hyperflexion of the neck.

ANSWERS

45-1. b. The thyroid cartilage lies at approximately the same level as the fourth cervical vertebra. Other landmarks include:
C1 level: Angle of the mandible
C3 level: Hyoid bone
C6 level: Cricoid cartilage.

45-2. a. The transverse process of the atlas is palpable in the region between the angle of the mandible and the mastoid process. The atlas contains no body; it is simply a bony ring. Diving accidents frequently are the cause of atlas fractures (also known as a Jefferson fracture).

45-3. d. Numbness in the fingers, decreased grip strength, and a diminished triceps tendon test are all signs of C7-C8 radiculopathy. Radiography of the cervical spine should be done, but there are only seven cervical vertebrae so a C8 fracture cannot exist.

45-4. b. The atlantoaxial joint accounts for about 50% of lateral rotational range in the neck. The remaining rotation is cumulative between the intravertebral joints.

45-5. d. Although all options listed are helpful, the teaching and enforcement of proper tackling technique and avoidance of "spearing" (using the helmet as a battering ram) are most effective in preventing cervical spine injury.

45-6. c. The next best step in this patient is to obtain flexion and extension views of the neck to evaluate for ligamentous instability without fracture. No assistance or manipulation of the neck should be given. The patient must initiate all motion as pain will serve to limit motion and prevent additional injury.

45-7. d. A computerized tomography scan of the neck is sometimes required to visualize fractures of first cervical vertebrae (atlas) not evident on plain films. One additional note: flexion and extension views are contraindicated in light of the patient's sobriety.

45-8. b. When the neck is flexed forward about 20 degrees, the natural lordotic posture is lost and the vertebrae are vertically aligned in a segmented column. An axial load in this position causes the force to be directed vertically through the vertebrae and the shock-absorbing muscular supports of the neck. Too large of an axial load in this position is the most frequent mechanism of cervical fractures and dislocations.

CHAPTER **46**

Fractures and Dislocation of the Cervical Spine

Evan S. Bass, MD

QUESTIONS

46-1. The most effective tool in preventing cervical spine injuries in football is:
   a. a thorough flexibility and strengthening program for the neck.
   b. use of a neck roll.
   c. use of a cowboy collar.
   d. enforcing proper tackling techniques.

46-2. A football player is seen 1 week after a traumatic neck injury, complaining of ongoing neck pain with motion. Lateral, anteroposterior, and open mouth views completed on the day of injury were normal. Neurological examination results are normal, and the only physical finding is lower cervical pain with motion. The physician should next:
   a. treat conservatively with antiinflammatory medication and range-of-motion exercises.
   b. repeat the cervical spine radiography series with oblique views.
   c. obtain flexion and extension lateral radiographs of the neck, allowing the patient to initiate motion of his neck to its full limitations of motion.

d. obtain flexion and extension lateral radiographs of the neck with the cervical spine carefully manipulated and positioned by the physician or technician.

46-3. A teenager is seen in the emergency department after diving from a cliff into shallow water. He is slightly inebriated and has tenderness behind the angle of the jaw and posterior occipital area. Lateral, anteroposterior, and open mouth odontoid views of the neck are all normal. Neurological examination results are normal. The physician should next:

a. order oblique view, plain radiography of the neck.

b. obtain flexion and extension lateral radiographs of the neck, allowing the patient to initiate motion of his neck to its full limitations of motion.

c. obtain flexion and extension lateral radiographs of the neck, with the cervical spine carefully manipulated and positioned by the physician or technician.

d. order a computerized tomography scan.

46-4. The most common mechanism of serious neck injury in football is:

a. axial loading with neck slightly extended.

b. axial loading with neck flexed slightly forward.

c. hyperextension of the neck.

d. hyperflexion of the neck.

ANSWERS

46-1. d. Although all options listed are helpful, teaching and enforcement of proper tackling techniques and avoidance of "spearing" (from using the helmet as a battering ram) represent the most effective measure in preventing cervical spine injury.

46-2. c. The physician should order flexion and extension radiography of the neck to evaluate for ligamentous instability without fracture. No assistance or manipulation of the neck is to be given for these films. The patient must initiate all motion as pain will serve to limit motion and prevent additional injury.

46-3. d. A computerized tomography scan of the neck is sometimes required to visualize fractures of first cervical vertebrae (atlas) not evident on plain radiographs. One additional note: flexion and extension views would be contraindicated here because of the patient's insobriety.

46-4. b. When the neck is flexed forward about 20 degrees, natural lordotic posture is lost and the vertebrae are vertically aligned in a segmented column. An axial load in this position causes the force to be directed vertically through the vertebrae and intervertebral disks, and the shock-absorbing muscular supports of the neck are lost. Too large an axial load in this position is the most frequent mechanism of cervical fractures and dislocation.

CHAPTER 47

Extraaxial Cervical Spine Injury

James M. Moriarity, MD

QUESTIONS

47-1. All of the following are considered contraindications to contact sports, EXCEPT:
   a. asymptomatic patient with radiographic evidence of spinal stenoses.
   b. an athlete with Down syndrome with an atlanto-dens measurement of 4.5 mm.
   c. an athlete with his second episode of transient quadriparesis.
   d. spear tackler's spine.

47-2. Signs of C5 radiculopathy include:
   a. diminished triceps reflex.
   b. weakness of ipsilateral trapezius.
   c. weakness of finger extension.
   d. weakness of shoulder abduction.

47-3. Cervical rotation is:
   a. greatest at C1-C2.
   b. greatest at C4-C5.
   c. equally distributed along the cervical spine.
   d. greatest at the atlantooccipital joint.

47-4. Nodding of the head primarily involves motion of:
   a. the lower cervical segments.
   b. the atlantoaxial joint.
   c. the atlantooccipital joint.
   d. the middle cervical segments.

47-5. Which of the following statements is false?
   a. the first cervical nerve exits in the C0-C1 occipital membrane.
   b. shoulder shrugging is a C4 nerve root action.
   c. the C5 nerve root exits at the C5-C6 disk space.
   d. wrist flexion is a C7 nerve root action.

ANSWERS

47-1. a. Asymptomatic patients discovered to have radiographic evidence of spinal stenoses based on Pavlov ratios should not be prohibited from contact sports. Although there is a theoretical increase in the possibility of incurring an episode of transient quadriparesis, radiographic measurements alone are not sufficient criteria to exclude participation. Patients with a history of two or more episodes of transient quadriparesis should be withheld from contact sports as should individuals with predisposing conditions that favor axial loading such as spear tackler's spine. Instability of the C1-C2 vertebrae is a contraindication to contact activity.

47-2. d. The C5 nerve root innervates the deltoid muscle, which participates in shoulder abduction. Trapezius innervation is C4, biceps reflex C6, triceps reflex C7, and finger extension C7-C8.

47-3. a. Cervical rotation is a function of the design of the C1-C2 vertebrae. The superior projection of the dens (odontoid) into the ring of the C1 vertebra permits cervical rotation. The taut transverse and alar ligament resists posterior displacement of the dens onto the spinal cord and maintains the atlanto-dens interval at <4 mm during flexion and extension motion.

47-4. c. Nodding of the head primarily occurs at the atlantooccipital joint with some contribution from the upper vertebrae. Nodding is a demonstration of upper cervical motion, whereas bowing demonstrates lower cervical motion.

47-5. c. There are eight pairs of cervical nerves, with the first pair exiting in the occipital membrane. The cervical nerve roots exit in the disk space above; the thoracic and lumbar nerve roots exit from the disk space below, with C8 exiting below C7 (above T1); C5 nerve root exits in the C4-C5 disk space. Accordingly, a C3-C4 herniated disk could be expected to affect C4 nerve root activity such as trapezius strength.

CHAPTER 48

Cervical Spine Injuries: On-Field Management

Andrew W. Nichols, MD

QUESTIONS

48-1. A left lateral blow to a football player's helmet by an opposing player results in a sudden rightward deviation of his head and neck. He does not lose consciousness and denies neck pain, although he develops acute left upper extremity aching and weakness (affecting multiple nerve root levels). His symptoms resolve completely within 10 minutes. The most likely injury this player has sustained is a(n):
   a. cervical ligament disruption.
   b. transient quadriparesis.
   c. "burner" or "stinger."
   d. spinal cord contusion.
   e. acute intervertebral disk herniation.

48-2. For which of the following isolated clinical situations would it be unnecessary to use full spinal precautions when transporting an injured contact sport player off the field?
   a. unilateral deltoid weakness that improves during the initial evaluation.
   b. confusion or abnormal mentation.
   c. cervical pain or tenderness.
   d. dysesthesias of the upper extremity that develop during active cervical range of motion.

48-3. A football player sustains a blow to the vertex of the helmet and is found to be lying unconscious on the field in the prone position. As the head and neck are manually stabilized by the team leader, the initial assessment reveals the airway, breathing, and circulation to be intact. The proper technique for transferring the injured player to a spine board for transport is to:

a. "log-roll" the player into the prone position onto the spine board while maintaining head and neck traction.

b. "log-roll" the player into the supine position in the direction away from the rescuers and onto the spine board while the team leader uses the "cross-arm" maneuver of head and neck stabilization.

c. "log-roll" the player into the supine position in the direction of the rescuers and onto the spine board while the team leader uses the "cross-arm" maneuver of head and neck stabilization.

d. "log-roll" the player into the supine position in the direction away from the rescuers without the team leader using the "cross-arm" maneuver of head and neck stabilization.

e. "log-roll" the player into the supine position in the direction of the rescuers without the team leader using the "cross-arm" maneuver of head and neck stabilization.

48-4. The appropriate time to remove a football helmet from an injured football player with a suspected cervical spine injury is:

a. on the field, before transfer to the spine board.

b. on the field, after transfer to the spine board.

c. in the hospital emergency room, so that radiographs of the cervical spine may be obtained.

d. in the hospital emergency room, after lateral cervical spine radiographs have been obtained and are confirmed to be negative.

48-5. Clinical characteristics that are consistent with cervical cord injury include all of the following, EXCEPT:

a. bilateral extremity symptoms.

b. unidermatomal involvement.

c. upper and lower extremity involvement.

d. positive Babinski response.

e. bowel and/or bladder dysfunction.

ANSWERS

48-1. c. A "burner" (or "stinger") results from an acute "stretch" or "impingement" injury to the brachial plexus due to forced lateral deviation of the head. The "stretch" type and "impingement" type injuries affect the upper extremity, which is respectively contralateral and ipsilateral to the direction in which the head is deviated. The common symptoms of a burner include *unilateral* upper extremity aching, burning, weakness, and numbness. Multiple nerve root levels may be affected, and symptoms typically resolve spontaneously. Cervical spine ligamentous disruption generally presents initially with neck stiffness alone. Transient quadriparesis is characterized by motor and/or sensory deficits, which are often *bilateral* and may affect the upper *and* lower extremities. Spinal cord contusion (burning hands syndrome) usually presents with *bilateral* upper extremity motor and/or sensory symptoms, without neck pain.

48-2. a. The presence of upper extremity motor weakness that improves rapidly in an alert individual in the absence of neck pain or tenderness, should not require the need for full cervical precautions during transport. The presence of abnormal mentation, cervical pain or tenderness, or the appearance of dysesthesias during active range of motion indicate that full spinal precautions should be undertaken prior to transport.

48-3. c. The player with a suspected cervical spine injury should be transferred by the "log-roll" maneuver directly onto the spine board into the supine position for transport. The "cross-arm" maneuver allows the rescuer stabilizing the head and neck to maintain better cervical spine traction as the arms "unwind" during the turn process from prone to supine. The injured player should be "log-rolled" *toward* the rescuers, who are stationed at the shoulders, knees, and hips.

48-4. d. The football helmet should be left in place in the case of suspected cervical spine injury until the player has been transported to an equipped emergency facility and after cervical spine radiographs, which may be obtained with the helmet in place, are interpreted as negative for fracture. If airway, respiratory, or circulatory compromise is present, it is usually possible to adequately access the face to perform rescue maneuvers by removing the helmet face mask. This is best achieved by using a knife blade to cut the plastic loops that fasten it to the shell and flipping the face mask superiorly. Alternatively, if an older style face mask that does not have plastic loops is used, boltcutters may be used to remove the face mask. The helmet, when left in place, is useful to achieve immobilization by anchoring the head to the spine board with lightweight bolsters and tape. If for some reason the helmet must be removed prior to radiological cervical spine clearance, it should be removed only by personnel who are trained in the proper technique, as excessive jostling during removal may lead to further damage to an unstable cervical spine. The proper technique of removal calls for two individuals: one who stabilizes the chin and the other who stabilizes the helmet. After the cheek pads are removed, the person stabilizing the helmet spreads the helmet laterally and pulls longitudinally to extract the helmet. New proprietary devices are now available for easily removing helmets.

48-5. b. Involvement of a single dermatome is characteristic of a nerve root injury. Injury to the spinal cord often produces bilateral neurological symptoms that involve both upper and lower extremities, are associated with long tract signs, and bowel or bladder dysfunction.

C H A P T E R **49**

Low Back Pain

Murray E. Allen, MD

Robert J. Johnson, MD

QUESTIONS

49-1. Among gymnasts, defects at the pars interarticularis have been observed at an incidence of:
   a. 5%.
   b. 10%.
   c. 20%.
   d. 30%.
   e. 40%.

49-2. Which statement on risk factors for low back pain is **true**?
   a. overall, low back pain is an old person's disorder, commonest after age 50.
   b. short, fat persons have a high incidence of low back pain.
   c. good posture can prevent low back pain.
   d. unfitness is a risk factor for low back pain.
   e. low back pain is a physical disorder; psychological factors play a minor role.

49-3. Which treatment for low back pain is counterproductive and therefore **not indicated**?
   a. exercise, including back extensions.
   b. education and psychosocial support/advice.

    c. encouragement to early return to work/sports before 100% cured.

    d. bedrest, usually for 2 weeks in the beginning.

    e. avoiding analgesic/relaxant drugs.

49-4. In defects of the pars interarticularis, spondylolisthesis, which is true?

    a. the pars develops a stress fracture, which overheals at the site with body elongation of the pars, "pushing" the vertebral body forward.

    b. the pars develops a fracture, which becomes unstable, allowing the vertebral body to "slip" forward.

49-5. Disk surgery may be indicated:

    a. in low back pain with protruded disk as seen on myelogram, computerized tomography scan, or magnetic resonance imaging.

    b. in low back pain with significant degeneration of the disk at one level.

    c. in radiculopathy with progressive neurological deficit.

    d. in prolonged incapacitating low back pain with positive imaging study.

ANSWERS

49-1. b. About 10% of all sporting injuries occur to the low back; knees are overall most common of the serious injuries. Among gymnasts, low back pain is very common, and about 10% of females have verified symptomatic pars interarticularis defects, probably related to repeated compression-extension strains.

49-2. d. Common risks are unfitness, age 20s, possibly tall and fat, smoking, workplace stresses, and psychological issues. Neutral factors are sex and obesity (apart from fitness level). Major positive factors for chronic back complaints are psychosocial stability, lack of somatization, and work satisfaction.

49-3. d. Rest promotes atrophy of healthy tissues and increased atrophy of injured tissues and should be avoided in patients with low back pain. The overload principle also applies to the low back. Treatment should consist of exercise, education, psychosocial advice, return to early work before cure, and avoidance of analgesic and relaxant drugs.

49-4. a. The mechanisms for the appearance of forward override of one vertebral body over the lower one, in spondylolisthesis, is probably an overgrowth of the pars' stress fracture, which overgrows in the youth, resulting in a "push" effect upon the vertebral body. An acute slip of the vertebral body can occur, usually with very extreme shearing forces to the low back and a very dramatic acute cauda equina syndrome, which is a surgical emergency. This is very rare.

49-5. c. All imaging studies have false-positive rates of over 30%. The mere presence of a disk bulge may be unassociated with any symptoms. Surgery should not be performed for low back pain per se. It is indicated in cauda equina syndrome, radiculopathy with progressive neurological deficit, and recurrent radiculopathy with persistent neurological deficits. All of these indications should prompt an imaging study to confirm the clinical side (left or right) and level of pathology. If all these provisos are not met, then nonsurgical approaches have a higher success rate overall.

CHAPTER 50

Spondylolysis and Spondylolisthesis

Peter G. Gerbino II, MD

Lyle J. Micheli, MD

QUESTIONS

50-1. The single most frequent cause of chronic low back pain in the young athlete is:
   a. muscle strain.
   b. infection.
   c. spondylolysis.
   d. herniated disc.

50-2. Spondylolysis in the young athlete is:
   a. a congenital malformation of the vertebral posterior elements.
   b. a stress fracture caused by cyclic loading.
   c. a condition that only occurs in elite athletes.
   d. treated by restriction of activity.

50-3. Spondylolisthesis:
   a. is progressive and painful.
   b. is treated by spinal fusion.
   c. is usually the source of chronic back pain when found in adults.
   d. means "vertebral sliding."

50-4. Plain radiographs:
   a. can allow measurement of percent slip.
   b. show the pars damage in all cases.

  c. can be used to predict symptoms.

  d. should be avoided in young people.

50-5. Treatment of spondylolysis and spondylolisthesis in athletes:
  a. always involves rigid bracing.
  b. can usually be done with activity modification and physical therapy.
  c. always results in bony union.
  d. has been proven to be accelerated by the use of bone stimulators.

50-6. A young elite level gymnast presents at your office; she has been having back pain for the last few months, which prevents her from competing. There was no acute injury to initiate her symptoms; they started insidiously. It hurts most during the back walkover, which causes a deep burning in the low back for the next several hours. There is a constant background of ache. A few days out of the gym and she feels only slightly improved, but one back walkover and the pain returns. The pain is low in the back, close to the midline. There are no radiations anywhere, not to buttocks or legs. She has no reflex, sensory, or motor alterations in her legs; straight leg raising is normal. There is no hint of other joint problems, and no arthritis in her family history. What is your provisional diagnosis?
  a. psychological; she may be looking for a honorable exit from the sport.
  b. sacroiliitis, the beginning of a possible seropositive arthritis, maybe ankylosing spondylitis.
  c. facet joint sprain.
  d. diskogenic pain, possibly an early disk prolapse.
  e. stress fracture across the pars interarticularis, part of spondylolisthesis, with or without any anterior realignment of the vertebra.

50-7. With the young gymnast above, what is the laboratory test that will most likely clinch your diagnosis, although it might not be the first test ordered?
  a. routine spine radiography.
  b. technetium 99m nuclear bone scan, especially with the single photon emission computerized tomography (SPECT) views.
  c. Computerized axial tomography scan of low back.
  d. HLA-B27 antigen test.
  e. Diskogram.

50-8. A 14-year-old male hockey player was treated for mild (grade 1) spondylolisthesis and has been playing hockey without symptoms for the past year. His parents want another opinion concerning whether he should have any restrictions from contact sports because of his findings. Recent radiographs again showed the grade 1 spondylolisthesis. The current recommendations would be:
  a. no collision sports.
  b. no contact sports.

c. no restrictions.

d. no running sports.

50-9. A highly competitive 13-year-old female basketball player with low back pain is found to have unilateral spondylolysis of L5 on plain radiography, and a technetium 99m bone scan shows marked uptake in the same abnormal region as on the radiograph. The best recommendation for this athlete is that she:

a. may play basketball as long as she is pain-free and without medication.

b. may play basketball if wearing a thoracolumbosacral orthosis and taking nonsteroidal antiinflammatory drugs.

c. should be sidelined from all sports until the lesion has healed as seen on the bone scan.

d. should be sidelined from all sports for 1 year after the lesion has healed.

ANSWERS

50-1. c. Low back pain in young people is much less common than in adults. While most adult low back pain is diskogenic, most young athlete low back pain is spondylolytic.*

50-2. b. Pars interarticularis fracture or defect has never been found congenitally. Repeated hyperextension is felt to cause pars overload and stress fracture. Any athlete can develop spondylolysis. Virtually any sport can be played in the brace symptom-free.

50-3. d. Spondylolisthesis is rarely progressive and frequently not painful. Fusion is reserved for those rare cases that do not respond to conservative therapy. In adults with spondylolisthesis, degenerative disk pain, facet arthropathy pain, or spinal stenosis pain, may cause low back pain. The Greek roots "spondylos" and "olisthein" mean "vertebra" and "to slip" respectively.

50-4. a. Reliance on plain radiographs will frequently miss a fine spondylolysis stress fracture. Only SPECT bone scan can identify a pre-spondylolytic stress reaction. Trying to avoid excess radiation in any patient is laudable but may result in failure to diagnose this condition. Percent slip and slip angle can easily be measured on standing lateral radiographs.

50-5. a. In athletes bracing will always be required to prevent hyperlordosis if the sport is to be continued. Activity modification and physical therapy will help but do not provide adequate support to the overstressed spine. Bony union is a goal of therapy but is not necessary to achieve the pain-free state. Bone stimulators may provide some benefit, but no controlled studies have been done.

50-6. e. This is a typical case history of a young female athlete with symptomatic spondylolisthesis. Note that the word "slip" is not used in the answer, although this word is commonly used to express the anterior realignment of the superior vertebra on the one below. The current concept is that the stress fracture of the pars overgrows, a not uncommon event in fractures in youngsters, and this overgrowth lengthens the pars (it is a long bone, with a joint at each end). From a biomechanical perspective, the increased pars length would "push" the superior vertebral body anteriorly. This is not a "slip"; however, the word "push" will probably not catch on.

50-7. b. Routine spine radiography will spot the so-called slip but may miss the diagnosis. The SPECT scan is the most accurate but may not be necessary. In an athlete with typical clinical findings and a minor slip on radiography, your management will probably be the same, with or without the bone scan.

*Miki T et al: Congenital laminar defect of the upper lumbar spine associated with pars defect. A report of eleven cases, *Spine* 16(3):353-355, 1991.

50-8.   c. The incidence of spondylolisthesis reaches its peak at age 10, and after this age the incidence levels off. Therefore, from the epidemiological perspective, most cases of spondylolisthesis had their start before age 10 and it is discovered later. An asymptomatic 14 year old probably has had the problem for many years and is stable. This patient can be treated as if normal.

50-9.   a. Actually, the scan will more likely be positive on both sides, even though radiography may suggest that the problem is unilateral. The key in this patient is the back pain; then there is the assumption that it is coming from the spondylolisthesis until proven otherwise. Therefore treat as spondylolisthesis, and restrict activity according to symptoms. The use of a good back brace may help restrict her back extension, limit repetitive pars stress, and help her keep partially active, as long as she is back pain–free with the activity.

CHAPTER 51

Lumbar Spine Pain: Rehabilitation and Return to Play

Andrew J. Cole, MD, FACSM

Stanley A. Herring, MD, FACSM

QUESTIONS

51-1. The initial program of exercise for acute low back pain should be:
   a. only flexion.
   b. only extension.
   c. both.
   d. neither.

51-2. The single best predictor of a new injury during athletic activity is:
   a. inadequate warm-up.
   b. history of previous injury.
   c. type of playing surface used.
   d. participation in a contact sport.

51-3. Physical modalities for treatment of lumbar spine pain:
   a. are best used alone.
   b. are best used in combination with other physical modalities.
   c. are best used in combination with other physical modalities, education, medication, manual therapy, mechanical therapy, and therapeutic exercise.
   d. are best used in combination with therapeutic exercise only.

51-4. Following an uncomplicated low back sprain in an athlete, one of the following is probably the best advice:
  a. complete bedrest for at least 4 weeks.
  b. complete bedrest for about 2 weeks.
  c. complete bedrest for 2 days.
  d. lie down briefly and do a few gentle floor exercises when the pain is bad, but otherwise attempt to conduct activities as close as possible to usual.
  e. return to play and usual training program right away.

ANSWERS

51-1. d. The initial program of exercise should be based on the initial assessment, reproducible patterns of painful motion, and presumed pathology. If the athlete's pain decreases and/or centralizes with repeated flexion, this would be the initial neutral spine bias. If repeated extension decreases and/or centralizes the pain, this would be the initial neutral spine bias. Since acute lumbar spine pain usually limits range of motion more in one plane than the other, choice c is incorrect. Choice d is correct since the most comfortable neutral bias is chosen based on the initial assessment, reproducible patterns of painful movement, and presumed pathology—*either* flexion or extension bias may therefore be chosen, but not necessarily by arbitrary exclusion of other exercise.

51-2. b. While a variety of intrinsic and extrinsic factors have been analyzed to predict who will become injured, the single best predictor for a new injury during sporting activity is the history of a previous injury.

51-3. c. Choice d is incomplete since manual therapy, soft tissue and myofascial techniques, and mobilization help optimize soft tissue and articular function so that therapeutic exercise can train muscles and posture at their optimal position of function. Recent research has shown that passive modalities have no benefit in the management of low back or neck injuries.

51-4. d. Rest does not facilitate healing of back strains. Recent studies have shown that in a group of acutely injured persons, those that did the best were in the group told to return to work with no time off and no bedrest. The rested groups did poorly. Previous research found that 2 days of rest was better than 2 weeks, but now it appears that even less rest is the best.

C H A P T E R **52**

Knee Anatomy and Mechanisms of Injury

David V. Anderson, MD

QUESTIONS

52-1. Contact hyperextension injury is most likely to result in damage to which structure?
   a. posterior cruciate ligament (PCL).
   b. anterior cruciate ligament (ACL).
   c. patella.
   d. posterior horn of medial meniscus.

52-2. During sports, posterior cruciate injuries are most likely associated with an injury to what other structure?
   a. ACL.
   b. medial meniscus.
   c. articular cartilage.
   d. lateral meniscus.

52-3. Loss of which ACL function is associated with increased stress on the posterior horn of the meniscus?
   a. varus/valgus restraint.
   b. external rotation restraint.
   c. control of femoral glide during flexion/extension.
   d. hyperextension control.

52-4. Lateral collateral ligament (LCL) tears:
   a. are second only to ACL tears in athletes.
   b. occur secondary to contact valgus stress.
   c. are common but frequently overlooked.
   d. are uncommon.

52-5. Articular damage to the patella occurring with dislocations is usually due to:
   a. avulsions.
   b. contact with the lateral femoral condyle at the time of reduction.
   c. contact with the dislocation, producing force.
   d. bipartite patella.

ANSWERS

52-1. a. Hyperextension mechanisms can result in damage to many structures including the PCL and the posterior lateral complex; the ACL is taut in extension and is less likely to tear first, for with continued extension the tibia usually translates posteriorly and ACL tension is reduced.

52-2. c. Although the most frequent cause of PCL injuries in general is violent contact associated with motor vehicle accidents, causing a wide range of injuries to multiple ligaments and cartilage, as well as neurovascular structure, "isolated" PCL injuries are more likely associated with articular surface damage in contrast to meniscal damage seen with ACL tears.

52-3. c. The posterior horns of the meniscus cradle the posterior femoral condyles during flexion. With anterior tibial translation due to normal mechanics as well as quadriceps pull, these structures are even more stressed unless that translation is restrained by an intact ACL. Increased internal rotation as well as loss of femoral meniscal kinematics from hyperextension also put the menisci at risk.

52-4. d. The proportionate occurrence of ligament injuries is: ACL > MCL > ACL/MCL > PCL > LCL. ACL accounts for about half of knee ligament injuries, and MCL about one-fourth.

52-5. b. The medial facet of the patella or, less commonly, the lateral femoral condyle often sustains at least articular surface damage if not fractures secondary to the stress of the reduction if not the dislocation. Bipartite fragments are typically superolateral in location and may infrequently be the source of fracture fragments secondary to avulsions or incidental anatomical findings.

CHAPTER 53

Knee Ligament Injuries

James G. Garrick, MD

QUESTIONS

53-1. The primary role of the anterior cruciate ligament (ACL) is:
   a. to control rotation at the knee.
   b. to limit forward excursion of the tibia.
   c. to limit backward excursion of the tibia.
   d. to limit hyperextension.

53-2. The most common mechanism of injury for an ACL sprain is:
   a. hyperextension of the knee.
   b. hyperflexion of the knee.
   c. a blow to the medial aspect of the knee.
   d. a cutting or deceleration maneuver.

53-3. Which of the following symptoms would *not* suggest a sprain of the ACL?
   a. a "pop" or "snap."
   b. something "slipping out of place."
   c. swelling.
   d. locking.

53-4. Which of the following is *least* true regarding sprains of the posterior cruciate ligament?
   a. less common than sprains of the ACL.
   b. the result of a blow to the anterior tibia.
   c. associated with a positive posterior drawer test.
   d. more frequent in sports than ACL sprains.

53-5. Which of the following is the most reliable test for continuity of the ACL?
   a. magnetic resonance imaging.
   b. anterior drawer test.
   c. Lachmann test.
   d. arthrogram.

53-6. Which of the following activities is *least* likely to be associated with sprains of the ACL?
   a. alpine skiing.
   b. basketball.
   c. figure skating.
   d. soccer.

53-7. Lachmann's test is conducted with the knee flexed at:
   a. 0-15 degrees.
   b. 20-39 degrees.
   c. 40-59 degrees
   d. 60-89 degrees.
   e. 90 degrees.

53-8. A grade II sprain of the medial collateral ligament knee of an adolescent athlete is best treated by:
   a. immobilization in a cast.
   b. immobilization in a brace.
   c. mobilization in a hinged knee brace.
   d. mobilization in a Palumbo brace.

53-9. An acute "isolated" 3-degree tear of the ACL is clinically best demonstrated by a(an):
   a. anterior drawer sign.
   b. pivot shift.
   c. Lachmann's test.
   d. abduction stress test at 30 degrees of flexion.
   e. abduction stress test at 0 degrees.

53-10. The anterior drawer test for anterior cruciate laxity may be negative due to:
   a. hamstring spasm.
   b. knee flexed at 90 degrees.
   c. proprioceptive inhibition.
   d. apprehension positive.
   e. quadriceps spasm.

53-11. In an acute hemarthrosis that followed a valgus rotation injury of the knee, approximately what percent have sustained a partial or complete ACL tear?
   a. 0%.
   b. 25%.
   c. 50%.
   d. 75%.
   e. 100%.

53-12. A 19-year-old male football player had a major reconstruction of a torn ACL plus a medial meniscectomy. The most important muscle(s) for stabilization and protection of the ACL ligament is/are:
   a. gastrocnemius.
   b. hip flexors.
   c. quadriceps.
   d. hamstrings.
   e. posterior tibialis.

53-13. As the team doctor, you attended a field athlete who was struck to the ground, his knee "valgus" strained. He had never had any knee problems in the past. He did not hear any "pop," nor did he think anything "gave way." He had some tenderness, which was maximum just above and below the medial joint line; the tenderness was not over a wide area but did include the medial joint line. There was only a subtle hint of soft tissue swelling in the area. The joint had a full and uncatching range of motion, although it was somewhat tender medially at full forced flexion and with a firm valgus stress, which did not cause the joint to open up. You were confident that there was no evidence of ligament laxity of ACL or PCL or collaterals, although he was large and muscular. There was no hint of joint effusion; you declined to attempt a joint tap. He did not object to this vigorous physical examination. What do you put down as your initial diagnosis?
   a. anterior cruciate ligament tear until proven otherwise.
   b. posterior ligament tear; it's harder to spot and should be at the top of the list.
   c. chondrocartilaginous injury; he will probably require arthroscopy later.
   d. medial capsular ligament and medial collateral third-degree sprain but not the triad.
   e. first-degree medial knee sprain.

ANSWERS

53-1.   c. The anatomy of the ACL runs from the anterior tibial tubercle on the tibia posteriorly and superiorly to just behind the lateral femoral condyle. This prevents the femur from translating backward or the tibia from translating forward.

53-2.   d. The ACL can be injured with valgus-type blows or strains, which can occur during cutting or deceleration maneuvers. When rapidly decelerating, such as in falls, or shifting back on one's ski bindings, the ACL can be under high loads.

53-3.   d. ACL injuries can snap, pop, and feel like something has slipped, and they swell, usually with a hemarthrosis, but they rarely jam the joint.

53-4.   d. Posterior cruciate ligament sprains are less common than ACL sprains.

53-5.   a. The MRI is the new gold standard, which is reliable independent of clinical limitations. The Lachmann test is the best clinical test, conducted at about 20° of knee flexion; in good hands it is more sensitive than the anterior drawer test. Both require a good feel of the endpoint, which in an ACL tear is a soft endpoint. In all clinical tests the combination of swelling, pain, spasm, and hemarthrosis can mask the tests.

53-6.   c. Note that figure skating is the only sport that does not pin the foot to the ground, an unfortunate method for tearing the ACL. During a fall with the foot pinned down, the full weight of the upper body can apply force upon the knee.

53-7.   a. Many think Lachmann's test is conducted somewhat like an anterior drawer test, but Lachmann described it at only 15 degrees. When translating the tibia anteriorly with this test, there should also be a soft endpoint.

53-8.   c. Recent studies in animals find the recovery time fastest and most complete in those who have been mobilized early. Movement (not rest) facilitates faster and more complete ligament repair.

53-9.   c. Lachmann's test performed properly is the most sensitive test.

53-10.   a. The hamstrings also prevent anterior displacement of the tibia, and in an apprehensive patient they can spasm easily. Pain also begets spasm.

53-11.   d. The ACL tear scenario with hemarthrosis will likely engender a tear about 75% of the time. If you see this scenario with hemarthrosis, think ACL tear until proven otherwise.

53-12.   d. Hamstrings are important to help stabilize the ACL-deficient motion. However, the hamstrings do not always automatically activate when they should for ACL protection. Therefore do not rely upon them entirely—the surgery is very helpful.

53-13.   e. You could be wrong with this innocent diagnosis, so you would want to follow up on it. But the minor findings and very focal point tenderness do not sound like major problems. This is a very common scenario of a minor knee sprain.

CHAPTER **54**

Meniscal Injuries

James G. Garrick, MD

QUESTIONS

54-1. Which of the following is *not* a function of the menisci?
   a. enhance nutrition of the articular cartilage.
   b. redistribute forces across the knee joint.
   c. contribute to stability of the knee.
   d. none of the above.

54-2. A meniscus tear would be *most* likely to occur in combination with injury to the:
   a. medial collateral ligament.
   b. lateral collateral ligament.
   c. anterior cruciate ligament.
   d. posterior cruciate ligament.

54-3. Which of the following would be *least* likely to be associated with an acute meniscus tear?
   a. rotational movement.
   b. weight bearing at moment of injury.
   c. "popping" or "snapping" sensation.
   d. a blow to the medial aspect of the knee.

54-4. Which of the following is *least* likely to be of historical significance in an acute tear of the medial meniscus?
 a. associated "pop" or "snap."
 b. immediate locking (inability to fully extend knee).
 c. preexisting chondromalacia of the patella.
 d. swelling (effusion).

54-5. Which of the following is the *most* reliable means of detecting the presence of a meniscus tear?
 a. magnetic resonance imaging.
 b. McMurray test.
 c. joint line tenderness.
 d. standing anteroposterior radiography.

54-6. Appropriate management of a meniscus tear includes:
 a. surgical repair (suture).
 b. excision of torn segment.
 c. rehabilitation and observation.
 d. all of the above.

54-7. Which of the following athletes is *most* likely to suffer a displaced bucket handle tear of the medial meniscus?
 a. a 55-year-old tennis player.
 b. a 23-year-old marathon runner.
 c. a 19-year-old soccer player.
 d. a 16-year-old swimmer.

ANSWERS

54-1. a. The menisci help to balance and evenly distribute the forces across the joint margin of the knee; they also contribute to stability, but they are not nutrient enhancers.

54-2. c. A force severe enough to tear the anterior cruciate ligament could also injure the meniscus, especially the medial meniscus. Medial collateral injuries can also be associated with meniscus injuries along the margin of the joint but can more commonly be isolated ligament sprains.

54-3. d. A blow to the medial aspect of the knee can sprain the lateral or opposite collateral ligament but probably not the medial ligament, which would most likely suffer only a focal bruise or less consequence.

54-4. c. Chondromalacia patella is a patellar problem; it can exist independent of meniscal injuries and does not make such injuries more vulnerable. Note that all the other options are in fact meniscal related.

54-5. a. The clinical tests of meniscal injuries are often associated with false-negative findings, so magnetic resonance imaging is becoming the most reliable indicator of meniscal injury.

54-6. d. Meniscal injuries have many approaches; all are appropriate, depending on the specifics of each injury.

54-7. c. The bucket handle tear requires a high weight-bearing load; the 55-year-old tennis player is probably not able to produce such high loads, the marathoner runs a straight line and is not likely to fall with another person on top of them, and the swimmer is non–weight bearing. This leaves the young soccer player at risk.

CHAPTER 55

Anterior Knee Pain and Overuse

J. Michael Wieting, DO, MEd

Douglas B. McKeag, MD, MS

QUESTIONS

55-1. Chronic recurring anterior knee pain:
   a. is always due to pathology involving the patella.
   b. may affect as many as 75% of all athletes.
   c. is a multifactorial problem with chronic overloading as a dominant factor.
   d. is caused by chronic hamstring weakness.
   e. is more common in males.

55-2. An important principle to remember when evaluating chronic recurring anterior knee pain is:
   a. diagnosis can usually be reliably made with plain radiography.
   b. erythrocyte sedimentation rate, complete blood count, liver function tests, and antibody testing are usually an essential part of the workup.
   c. ligamentous laxity is a factor in evaluation.
   d. physical examination should include assessment of gait and posture.

55-3. Treatment of anterior knee pain:
   a. is rarely successful without a specific identifiable cause.
   b. should include maintenance of usual activity level.

c. is usually straightforward after a careful history and physical examination.

d. is surgical in nature if conservative therapy does not produce satisfactory outcome in 3 months.

e. may involve management of leg-knee malalignments such as genu valgus, patellar tracking, or foot hyperpronation.

55-4. Chondromalacia patella is:
a. an arthroscopic diagnosis.
b. a separation of subchondral bone and cartilage from another bone.
c. caused by contusive microtrauma or a sprain with resultant inherent ligamentous laxity.
d. causes peripatellar synovitis.

55-5. One of these tendons does *not* form the surroundings of the pes anserinus area:
a. semitendinosus.
b. semimembranosus.
c. sartorius.
d. popliteus.
e. gracilis.

55-6. Baker's cyst at the back of the knee may be an extension of the:
a. semimembranosus bursa.
b. semitendinosus bursa.
c. pes anserinus.
d. Hoffa fat pad.
e. popliteus tendon sheath.

55-7. A 15-year-old girl visited your office with knee pain. She had started a school running program, something new to her. She had never been very athletic. She first noted the knee pain for an hour or so after a run; then it would linger into the night and occasionally into the next day. At first she could continue running, but not now. There was no acute trauma. Examination of her knees showed nothing; full range of painless movement, no tenderness on palpation anywhere, ligaments intact, no cartilage clicks, no patellar apprehension, no subpatellar grating or pain, and no swelling or hint of effusion. She was reasonably muscled, but you did not perform any accurate strength test. When lying, her legs looked straight, but when standing she demonstrated genu valgum with "squinting" patellae. The rear foot heel counter of her running shoes appeared to lean medially. What is your clinical diagnosis?
a. chondromalacia patellae.
b. patellofemoral pain syndrome.
c. iliotibial band friction syndrome.
d. popliteus tendinitis.
e. Osgood-Schlatter disease.

55-8. Besides overuse, what is the likely underlying etiology of the above girl's knee pain?
   a. chondrocartilage degenerative fibrillation under the patellar facets.
   b. foot hyperpronation motion causing knee rotation stress.
   c. knobbly knees with irritation of the fascia over the lateral femoral condyle.
   d. weakness of the posterior knee joint stabilizer muscle-tendon unit.
   e. inflammation of the tibial apophysis.

55-9. "Jumper's knee" has pain at which location?
   a. upper superior pole of patella.
   b. medial inferior to patella.
   c. lateral to patella, along the retinaculum.
   d. lateral to patella, but overlying the lateral femoral condyle.
   e. overlying the patellar tubercle and lower patellar tendon.

ANSWERS

55-1. c. Anterior knee pain is a complex, multifactorial problem, the dominant factor of which is chronic overloading. Occasionally it is due to patellar pathology. Anterior knee pain has been estimated to affect as many as 25% of all athletes. Hamstring weakness is generally not a factor in anterior knee pain. Additionally, anterior knee pain is more common in females. Malalignment factors in such knees are very common.

55-2. d. Although plain radiography views are the initial radiographic studies that would be done in the evaluation of anterior knee pain, a diagnosis should not be based solely on radiographic findings. These views would be valuable mostly in acute trauma or patellar alignment. Laboratory studies such as erythrocyte sedimentation rate, liver functions, and antibody testing as well as complete blood count would be obtained only if systemic inflammatory or metabolic disease was suspected. Ligamentous laxity can be a causative factor in anterior knee pain and should therefore be a key part of its evaluation. Bone scanning should be judiciously used if knee pain symptoms are prolonged (>3-4 months), diagnosis is uncertain, or pain limits activities of daily living.

55-3. e. Malalignment factors in the leg combined with overuse is perhaps the most common finding associated with recurrent or chronic knee pain. Treatment should include modification of activity (moderating the pace if a person is very active or, in the case of an inactive person, starting with baseline exercising and advancing as tolerated). Correcting foot hyperpronation and variations on patellar bracing and taping may help. Surgical treatment should only be considered if nonsurgical treatment fails for a period of greater than six months or if there is an obviously surgically correctable lesion.

55-4. a. Chondromalacia patella by definition is an arthroscopic diagnosis. It is a softening of patellar articular cartilage featuring roughened or fibrillated appearance and is considered the end stage of cartilage degeneration. Osteochondritis dissecans is a separation of subchondral bone and cartilage from another bone. Hoffa's syndrome is caused by contusive microtrauma or sprain with resultant inherent ligamentous laxity. Chondromalacia patella can occasionally cause peripatellar synovitis.

55-5. d. The popliteus is at the posterior lateral aspect of the knee, not anterior medial, which is the location of all the other muscles as they converge at the pes anserinus. Bursitis is common here.

55-6. a. The semimembranosus bursa, sometimes called a Baker's cyst, can be connected to the knee joint through a posterior-medial connection. Persons with arthritis and effusion can have an overflow of the effusion into the semimembranosus bursa. In extreme cases it can even gravitate down between the gastrocnemius and soleus muscles to produce a very large synovial-bursal swelling in the calf.

55-7. b. This is a very typical story of the malaligned foot-leg with anterior medial knee pain. The key history is lack of trauma, insidious onset, worse late in or after activity, worse with straight long distance running, and almost nothing to find when examining the knee. However, malalignment factors will be noted starting from the foot upwards, including wide Q angles, valgus angled patellae, foot hyperpronation, and a hyperpronating knee valgus stress during running or jumping.

55-8. b. Studies have shown that these common knee pains are usually associated with leg malalignment factors, the foot hyperpronation being the most common finding.

55-9. a. Jumpers, like basketball and volleyball players, will get a peculiar pain at the top of the patella, worse right at the moment of jumping as a sharp pain. Rest gives relief. It is probably an enthesopathy, like lateral epicondylitis, caused by repeated tension strains with microtears.

CHAPTER **56**

Rehabilitation of the Injured Knee

David B. Richards, MD

W. Benjamin Kibler, MD

QUESTIONS

56-1. The most important aspect of rehabilitating the injured athlete's knee is:
  a. returning to competition as soon as possible.
  b. decreasing pain and swelling.
  c. assessing for neurovascular injury.
  d. restoring normal knee function.

56-2. Rehabilitation of the injured knee is best accomplished through the use of which of these techniques?
  a. weight training.
  b. cycling and aerobic exercise.
  c. proprioceptive and sport-specific drills.
  d. all of the above.

56-3. Progression through the rehabilitation program is primarily dependent on which of the following?
  a. pain threshold of the athlete.
  b. meeting the specific criteria for progression at each phase of the program.
  c. the urgency with which the athlete needs to return to play.
  d. lack of symptoms.

ANSWERS

56-1. d. The top priority in the treatment and rehabilitation of the injured knee should be to restore that knee to normal function. Reducing pain and swelling are an important part of the acute phase of rehabilitation. Neurovascular status should be determined at the time of the injury and appropriate treatment rendered; problems here are uncommon. Although there may be significant external pressure to return athletes to competition (even from the athletes themselves), they must demonstrate near normal strength, range of motion, and performance on high speed sport-specific drills before they are allowed to return to play.

56-2. d. Proper rehabilitation is a multidisciplinary process involving modalities such as heat, ice, and electrical stimulation to help relieve the symptoms associated with the injury. It also utilizes weight training, aerobic and flexibility training. Lastly, as the patient progresses through a well-structured rehabilitation program, more sophisticated proprioceptive drills and sport-specific activities are utilized prior to returning to competition.

56-3. b. Progression through the rehabilitation program should be based on specific criteria established for each particular injury and modified according to individual patients needs. While a rehabilitation program may cause some discomfort, enduring great pain is not the objective. The need to return to play should never lead to "shortcuts" through the rehabilitation program. Resolution of pain symptoms is an early feature of the acute phase of injury rehabilitation.

CHAPTER **57**

Anatomy and Examination of the Hip

Carl Winfield, MD

QUESTIONS

57-1. The blood supply to the hip joint is best described as:
 a. very poor to the joint as a whole.
 b. limited blood supply to the femoral head itself.
 c. generous to the femoral head.
 d. generous to all portions except for the femoral neck.

57-2. To which area does hip joint pathology often refer pain?
 a. thoracic back.
 b. contralateral buttock.
 c. knee.
 d. umbilicus.

57-3. What physical sign or signs suggest a possible flexion contracture of the hip?
 a. Patrick's test (FABERE test).
 b. Gaenslen's test.
 c. Trendelenburg test.
 d. increased lumbar lordosis and Thomas test.

57-4. Which is a reliable method for detecting a true limb length discrepancy?
 a. measuring from the umbilicus to the medial malleolus.

b. measuring from the pubic tubercle to the lateral malleolus.

c. measuring from the anterior superior iliac spine to the medial malleolus.

d. measuring from the posterior superior iliac spine to the calcaneus.

e. radiography of feet, knees, hips with radiolucent measuring device.

57-5. The sacroiliac joint can be palpated by:

a. palpating 2 cm inferior to the posterior superior iliac spine.

b. palpating 5 cm superior to the ischial tuberosity.

c. palpating at the midpoint of the posterior superior iliac spine and the ischial tuberosity.

d. cannot be palpated.

ANSWERS

57-1. b. The vascular supply to the hip joint as a whole is generous. The femoral head is supplied by perforating capsular branches that derive from an extracapsular arterial ring, which is formed predominantly by the medial femoral circumflex artery with contributions from the lateral circumflex vessels. These form a reticular arterial system that runs along the neck of the femur, making the head extremely vulnerable to any trauma.

57-2. c. Pain involving the hip joint is often felt in the groin or medial thigh. However, with some disorders (e.g., Legg-Calvé-Perthes disease) up to 20% of patients may complain of knee pain only. Therefore it is always essential to evaluate the hip when a child complains of knee pain.

57-3. d. The Patrick or the FABERE (flexion, abduction, external rotation and extension) test is suggestive of sacroiliitis only in the absence of true hip joint pathology. A positive Gaenslen test is also suggestive of sacroiliitis. The Trendelenburg test is a result of pain in the weight-bearing hip or weakness of the ipsilateral gluteus medius muscle. Increased lordosis of the lumbar spine suggests the need to evaluate for flexion deformity of the hip, and the Thomas test will detect a hip flexion contracture. (Note: in most medical examinations, the use of proprietary names like Patrick or Thomas would not be used).

57-4. c. An erroneous leg length is measured from the umbilicus to the medial malleolus on both legs. Apparent leg length discrepancy may result from problems in pelvic obliquity or, as with scoliosis, problems of the lumbar spine. Leg length is often measured from the anterior superior iliac spine to the medial malleolus on the ipsilateral leg, but can also be affected by pelvic obliquity. The only truly accurate measure is spot radiography of feet, knees, and hips with a radiolucent measuring device. The other methods can be used for screening.

57-5. d. Because of the overhand of the ilium and the obstruction of the support ligaments, the sacroiliac joint is not directly palpable. It is only occasionally involved pathologically and even then it may be asymptomatic. Tenderness to palpation of the gluteal area may suggest sacroiliitis but is nonspecific. A positive Gaenslen test is suggestive of sacroiliitis. The Patrick (FABERE) test can suggest sacroiliitis only in the absence of true hip joint problems.

CHAPTER 58

Common Hip Injuries

Carl Winfield, MD

QUESTIONS

58-1. What is the most reliable diagnostic test for early detection of femoral neck stress fracture?
   a. physical examination.
   b. bone scan.
   c. radiography.
   d. observation.

58-2. What is the standard method of treatment of a quadriceps contusion in addition to rest and ice?
   a. immobilization with the knee in 120 degrees of flexion or more for at least the first 24 hours after injury.
   b. immobilization with the knee in full extension for the first 12 hours.
   c. continuous passive motion for the first 24 hours.
   d. aggressive stretching within the first 12 hours ("contract relax").

58-3. Which is *not* one of the four most common sites for an avulsion fracture of the hip/pelvis region?
   a. anterior superior iliac spine.
   b. inferior pubic ramus.
   c. ischial tuberosity.
   d. iliac crest.

58-4. Which of the following is *not* true of myositis ossificans?
   a. heterotopic bone should be surgically excised at the earliest possible moment after diagnosis.
   b. usually follows a deep contusion to a large muscle such as the quadriceps.
   c. the bony mass may shrink in size over a 3-6 month period.
   d. recurrent myositis ossificans may suggest a bleeding disorder.

58-5. What stretching exercises are most useful in treating piriformis syndrome?
   a. "hurdler's stretch."
   b. flexing, internally rotating, and adducting the hip.
   c. extending, externally rotating, and abducting the hip.
   d. slow, steady abduction with internal rotation.

58-6. "Meralgia paraesthetica" is an uncomfortable sensory neuropathy affecting the:
   a. forearm, a radial nerve palsy.
   b. dorsum of the foot, a peroneal nerve foot drop.
   c. calf, an adductor canal outlet neuropathy.
   d. thigh, a lateral femoral cutaneous nerve to the thigh neuropathy.
   e. axilla, from thoracic outlet syndrome.

ANSWERS

58-1. b. The history can be very suggestive in the endurance athlete, with a recent increase in training regimen being common. Radiographs may be negative early or may reveal periosteal new bone formation, endosteal thickening, or radiolucent line formation. A bone scan typically gives the diagnosis 2-8 days after the symptoms begin and is exceptionally sensitive in detecting femoral neck stress fractures.

58-2. a. Initial treatment of a quadriceps contusion involves immobilization in full knee flexion for the first 24 hours as well as ice; stretching the involved muscle would appear to be the principle. Active and passive range of motion exercises are then performed as well as progressive weight bearing as tolerated. Finally, stretching, strengthening, and proprioceptive exercises are instituted. After fully pain-free range of motion is achieved, noncontact sports may be resumed. If not treated properly and expeditiously, the athlete may have a prolonged recovery as well as an increased risk of developing myositis ossificans.

58-3. b. The true prevalence of avulsion fractures of the hip and pelvis is not known, as many are probably treated without being diagnosed. The four that are believed to be the most common are the anterior superior iliac spine, iliac crest, anterior inferior iliac spine, and ischial tuberosity. Other sites where avulsion fractures have been reported are the greater trochanter, lesser trochanter, and symphysis pubis. Avulsion fractures of the inferior pubic ramus have not been reported.

58-4. a. Heterotopic bone excision should not be performed prior to maturity of the lesion because recurrence will probably occur. Serial bone scans are recommended if maturity of the lesion is in question. Heat, ultrasound, deep massage, and aggressive range of motion should also be avoided in the early phase. Surgical excision is rarely indicated as recovery is usually complete and does not depend on resorption of the heterotopic bone.

58-5. b. The piriformis muscle originates from the anterior surface of the sacrum between the first and fourth sacral foramina. After passing through the greater sciatic foramen, it inserts on the upper surface of the greater trochanter of the femur. It acts as an external rotator of the hip. It is best stretched by flexing, internally rotating, and adducting the hip.

58-6. d. As it courses out from under the inguinal ligament near the anterior superior iliac spine, the lateral femoral cutaneous nerve to the thigh can be entrapped. It is only a sensory nerve, so no motor harm is ever done, although some patients panic and think they are paralyzed. This condition shows very definite sensory loss along the lateral thigh. In other cases numbish thighs without sensory loss can be present as a referred pain from pelvic or sacroiliac problems and can be confused for meralgia paraesthetica.

CHAPTER **59**

Ankle and Foot Anatomy

Aaron L. Rubin, MD

QUESTIONS

59-1. The largest bone in the foot is the:
   a. calcaneus.
   b. talus.
   c. navicular.
   d. cuboid.
   e. phalanx.

59-2. Medial ankle tenderness after an eversion injury would indicate possible injury to the:
   a. fibula.
   b. anterior talofibular ligament.
   c. peroneal tendon.
   d. deltoid ligament.
   e. calcaneofibular ligament.

59-3. The primary function of the tibialis anterior muscle is to:
   a. dorsiflex and supinate the foot.
   b. extend and dorsiflex the great toe.
   c. evert and plantarflex the foot.
   d. plantarflex and supinate the foot.
   e. none of the above.

59-4. The lateral column of the foot includes all the following bones, EXCEPT the:
   a. calcaneus.
   b. cuboid.
   c. fifth metatarsal.
   d. navicular.
   e. phalanges of fourth and fifth toes.

59-5. During the normal gait cycle for walking:
   a. the swing phase accounts for most of the cycle.
   b. there is a "double float phase" when neither foot is in contact with the ground.
   c. the stance phase accounts for about 60% of the cycle.
   d. the initial contact of the foot is with the forefoot.

ANSWERS

59-1. a. The calcaneus is the largest, strongest bone in the foot, making up the heel and most of the hindfoot.

59-2. d. The deltoid ligament is on the medial side of the ankle. The other structures listed are on the lateral side of the ankle.

59-3. a. The tibialis anterior is a primary dorsiflexor and supinator of the foot. The extensor hallucis longus, though in the same anterior compartment of the leg, extends and dorsiflexes the great toe. The peroneus brevis and longus in the lateral compartment of the leg evert and plantarflex the foot. The gastrocnemius and soleus in the superficial posterior compartment of the leg plantarflex and supinate the foot.

59-4. d. The navicular is part of the medial column of the foot, which also includes the calcaneus, talus, medial, and middle cuneiform and first and second metatarsals and phalanges. The middle column is made up of the lateral cuneiform, third metatarsal, and phalanx of the third toe. The calcaneus, cuboid, fourth and fifth metatarsals, and phalanx make up the lateral column.

59-5. c. The stance phase of contact with the foot on the ground is about 60% of the gait cycle. In walking, normal footstrike is with the heel and one foot is always in contact with the ground. The double float phase occurs in running, and in fact is a key definition of running when both feet are simultaneously off the ground—a disqualifier for race-walking.

CHAPTER 60

Ankle Ligament Injuries

Aaron L. Rubin, MD

QUESTIONS

60-1. The most commonly injured ligament by inversion-plantarflexion is the:
   a. calcaneofibular.
   b. posterior talofibular.
   c. anterior talofibular.
   d. deltoid.

60-2. The Ottawa ankle rules recommend radiography of the injured ankle if:
   a. there is bony tenderness of the malleolus.
   b. the athlete is unable to walk four steps at the time of injury.
   c. the athlete is unable to walk four steps at the time of examination.
   d. the athlete is older than 18.
   e. all of the above.

60-3. The fibular squeeze test is used to evaluate:
   a. lateral ankle sprains.
   b. navicular fractures.
   c. syndesmotic ankle sprains.
   d. Achilles tendon ruptures.

60-4. Instability of the deltoid ligament is evaluated by the:
   a. talar tilt.
   b. squeeze test.
   c. eversion stress test.
   d. anterior drawer test.

60-5. Initial management of ankle ligament sprains (first 24 hours) includes all, EXCEPT:
   a. rest.
   b. ice.
   c. compression.
   d. elevation.
   e. hot whirlpool.

60-6. In an athlete with an acute inversion sprain of the ankle, treatment emphasis should be placed on:
   a. immediate control of soft tissue swelling utilizing taping, wrapping, ice, and elevation.
   b. early ankle range of motion exercises to maintain near full ankle range of motion.
   c. strengthening exercises for the peroneals and tibialis posterior muscles.
   d. all of the above.
   e. none of the above; it should be casted.

60-7. A radiography-negative "pronation ankle sprain" that occurred during firm foot plant, slight foot dorsiflexion, and forced foot external rotation, characterized by swelling nearly to the knee, numbness over the dorsal foot, foot drop, and joint effusion, is most likely:
   a. third-degree complete anterior talofibular sprain.
   b. third-degree talofibular and talocalcaneal sprain.
   c. tibiofibular diastasis (syndesmosis disruption).
   d. early talar dome fracture.
   e. fracture of os trigonum.

60-8. For the pronation ankle sprain (above question), the underlying etiology of the foot drop and dorsal ankle/foot numbness is:
   a. swelling that reached the upper end of the interosseous membrane between the tibia and fibula and irritated the common peroneal nerve.
   b. concurrent injury to the lateral peroneal nerve.
   c. anterior compartment syndrome.
   d. posterior tibialis/soleus muscle compartment pressure.
   e. the cast was too tight.

60-9. A serious cause of persistent and progressive ankle pain and disability seen after a lateral inversion sprain that was initially expected to recover is:

a. peroneal tendinitis.

b. myositis ossificans.

c. osteomyelitis.

d. osteochondral injury of talar dome.

e. plantar fasciitis.

ANSWERS

60-1. c. The anterior talofibular is the most commonly injured ligament in the ankle. The mechanism is usually by inversion-plantarflexion. As the ankle continues to invert, the calcaneofibular and posterior talofibular may be affected. The deltoid is injured in eversion.

60-2. e. The Ottawa ankle rules were developed to avoid unnecessary radiographs in the emergency department for acute injuries. These should be considered a guideline and not replace clinical judgment.

60-3. c. The squeeze test helps in evaluating the distal tibia-fibula syndesmosis, although this injury is accompanied by major swelling, which makes the test a bit difficult. The calf squeeze test (Thompson test) is used to evaluate Achilles tendon ruptures. Palpation of the navicular and lateral ankle ligaments aids in diagnosis of injuries to these areas.

60-4. c. The eversion test aids in diagnosing instability of the deltoid ligament. The squeeze test helps diagnose syndesmotic injury. The anterior drawer and talar tilt tests are used to diagnose lateral ankle instability due to anterior talofibular tears.

60-5. e. The mnemonic "RICE" is used to remember rest, ice, compression, and elevation for the initial treatment of ankle sprains. Heat application should be avoided in initial management since it causes increased swelling and delays return to play. Recent advances in ankle sprain management include early active mobilization.

60-6. d. Old fashioned methods simply encouraged RICE. This is no longer enough by today's standards, which now include early range of motion exercises and strength training, starting about day 1. This can be started even in the grade 3 ankle sprains. This might seem aggressive, but it helps reduce the chance of adhesive joint disorders that are common following prolonged immobilization. Even third-degree sprains will heal and strengthen to normal with this approach, and those rare ones that become unstable can still be repaired surgically; the delay has been shown probably not to be harmful.

60-7. c. This is a major ankle sprain; if seen very early, it will be noted to have only anterior mortis line swelling, something not seen in other, more common ankle sprains. Shortly thereafter, this ankle becomes so swollen that landmarks become blurred.

60-8. a. The swelling can track up the interosseous membrane, reaching the common peroneal nerve at the back of the knee. Once out from around the knee, this nerve is out of the line of any inflammation from an ankle sprain, and yet it is the only nerve to control the foot drop and dorsal foot numbness. It can only be trapped at the back of the knee. A lot of injury is needed to track the swelling that high.

60-9. d. Watch out for the "simple" ankle sprain that is not. If it continues to swell and cause pain and grating that you did not expect, get another set of radiographs. The initial set may miss the talar dome fractures, but with some bone resorption at the fracture site, it will show up. If still concerned, order a computerized tomography scan, tomogram, or magnetic resonance imaging.

CHAPTER **61**

Ankle Fractures in Athletes
Angus M. McBryde, Jr., MD

QUESTIONS

61-1. A 12-year-old has a major ankle injury from a fall during a skate-board contest. Two years later tilt and shortening at the ankle joint are present. What was the original fracture?
   a. Tillaux fracture.
   b. triplane fracture.
   c. distal fibula epiphyseal injury.
   d. fracture of medial malleolus.
   e. Salter I distal tibia.

61-2. Generally good results from the surgical treatment of ankle fractures in athletes compared to the normal population are due to:
   a. better bone for healing.
   b. more aggressive rehabilitation programs available.
   c. better compliance in a sports medicine environment.
   d. all of the above.
   e. none of the above.

61-3. A 20-year-old has an ankle injury on the soccer field when he turns to the right sharply on a fixed pronated right foot. The fibula fracture would usually be:
   a. below the ankle.

b. above the ankle.
c. at level of ankle.
d. absent with only the tibia fractured.
e. comminuted.

61-4. A 15-year-old high-school cross-country runner has the onset of lateral ankle pain after a November meet; running causes pain and gait changes which are improved with rest. She could not remember the exact moment of onset. She is tender three finger breadths above the tip of the lateral malleolus. Anteroposterior, lateral, and oblique views of the ankle are negative at 5 days after injury. Further management at this point consists of:
  a. an air stirrup–type cast and reducing her running below the level of pain.
  b. Open reduction internal fixation (ORIF) of the distal fibular epiphyseal fracture.
  c. short leg cast for 6 weeks, then radiograph again for union of the fracture.
  d. foot and ankle taping and an emphasis on stretching and continued same level training and competition.
  e. cease all running and substitute with hiking.

61-5. The Danis-Weber classification system for ankle fracture:
  a. emphasizes the importance of anatomic fibular reduction.
  b. combines mechanism of injury with anatomic description.
  c. is not helpful in operative decision making.
  d. uses principles of external fixation.
  e. is not compatible with American Orthopaedic (AO) principles.

ANSWERS

61-1. b. Triplane fracture is a fracture with significant transepiphyseal fracture lines and displacement in several planes, which can interfere with continued normal physeal growth. Tillaux fracture, distal fibula epiphyseal injury, fracture of medial malleolus, and Salter I distal tibia fracture generally do not interfere substantially with epiphyseal growth and are rare causes of angulation or shortening in the lower extremity.

61-2. d. Athletes are generally younger with better bone stock. In the sports medicine environment, compliance, trainer and/or therapist monitoring, and established protocols permit quick return of motion, return of strength, and return of proprioceptive function.

61-3. b. The pronation external rotation injury generally causes a mortise/syndesmosis injury with medial failure, then lateral failure, and then a high fibular fracture. Fractures at and below the ankle joint have a different mechanism of injury. The same is true with tibial (medial malleolar usually) injury even with ligamentous sprain laterally. The above medial rotation mechanism in skiers can cause a "helicopter" fracture to the upper fibula; skiers who spin like a helicopter off a mogul are prone to this injury but due to tight ski boots, the lower fibula is saved, so it fractures higher up.

61-4. a. Fibula stress fracture is the probable diagnosis and is generally not at risk for major complication. Treatment consists of continued sports-specific stimulation while keeping it below the level that causes significant discomfort. Stress fracture can occur through the distal fibula epiphyseal region but is rare. Short leg cast and total elimination of running are rarely necessary.

61-5. a. AO classification does help with surgical decision making depending on the type of ankle fracture. It does not describe the mechanism of injury along with the anatomic description of the fracture. It does not use external fixation principles.

CHAPTER **62**

Rehabilitation of Ankle Injuries

Stephen M. Simons, MD

QUESTIONS

62-1. A biomechanical ankle platform system (BAPS or tilt) board is frequently used for ankle rehabilitation. What is the main purpose of
the BAPS board?
   a. increase muscle strength.
   b. increase range of motion.
   c. regain proprioception.
   d. improve flexibility.

62-2. The most appropriate therapy during the acute phase of ankle injury
for athletes is:
   a. full weight bearing with mild pain, ice, nonsteroidal antiinflammatory drugs (NSAIDs).
   b. rest, ice, compression, elevation.
   c. casting, NSAIDs.
   d. ice intermittently for 24 hours followed by heat the next 24
   hours.

62-3. Preventing ankle injury recurrence can sometimes be accomplished
with:
   a. taping.
   b. external supports (i.e., pneumatic or lace up).

    c. nothing protects against reinjury.

    d. high top shoes.

62-4. Which functional rehabilitation exercises are emphasized in the terminal phases?

    a. open kinetic chain with tubing and ankle weights.

    b. stretching with an inclined board.

    c. partial weight-bearing proprioception with BAPS board.

    d. closed kinetic chain exercises (i.e., foot on ground, full weight-bearing exercises).

    e. toe curls and marble pickups.

ANSWERS

62-1. c. A BAPS or tilt board may be used generally starting in the sub-acute phase of rehabilitation. This is often started in the partial weight-bearing position. These exercises are thought to improve the ligamentous position. Some more aggressive therapy clinics start range of motion and tilt board rehabilitation in the acute phase of some ankle sprains.

62-2. b. RICE (the acronym for rest, ice, compression, and elevation) is used during the acute phase. RICE should be used for the first 2-4 days. Some form of cryotherapy with elevation should be done 20 minutes every 2-3 hours. The ankle should be above the heart. Compression can dramatically decrease swelling. More recent additions to the RICE regimen include very early activation-mobilization routines.

62-3. b. External supports have proven helpful in preventing some re-injury. Tape quickly loses its support as exercise progresses. Both taping and external devices are better than no protection.

62-4. d. Successful ankle rehabilitation requires exercises and activities that begin to reproduce the sport demands. This can best be accomplished by closed kinetic chain (foot on the ground) exercises with full weight bearing.

C H A P T E R **63**

Sports Injuries to the Feet

Craig Wargon, DPM

QUESTIONS

63-1. The posterior tibial muscle:
   a. is an inverter and plantarflexor of the foot.
   b. is an inverter and dorsiflexor of the foot.

63-2. Treatment of calcaneal apophysitis can include the following, EXCEPT:
   a. heel lift.
   b. cryotherapy.
   c. functional custom orthotics.
   d. reassurance.

63-3. Degenerative changes within the Achilles' tendon are usually attributed to all, EXCEPT:
   a. partial rupture.
   b. aging process.
   c. vascular compromise within the tendon.
   d. chronic paratendonitis.

63-4. The following shoe recommendations are appropriate for a patient with heel pain syndrome (plantar fasciitis), EXCEPT:
   a. slightly higher heels.
   b. negative heel sandals.

c. shoes with thick midsoles.

d. shoes with good arch support or adjunctive arch supports.

63-5. Persistent heel valgus with single limb raise (standing on one foot with persistent long arch collapse) examination indicates:

a. calcaneal valgus.

b. posterior tibial tendon dysfunction.

c. tarsal coalition.

d. weak plantarflexors.

ANSWERS

63-1. a. The posterior tibial muscle has its primary insertion in the navicular tuberosity. It is an active inverter and plantarflexor of the foot. In stance it fires eccentrically to limit pronation of the foot and maintain the longitudinal arch. It is a major mover for springing forward at toe-off. Its origin along the lower one third posterior medial border of the tibia is also the common site of stress fractures in runners.

63-2. c. Calcaneal apophysitis (Sever's disease) is a common self-limiting condition in young athletes. It may represent osteochondrosis of the calcaneal apophysis. Radiographic examination demonstrates a dense calcaneal apophysis with or without fragmentation. Treatment consists of relative rest, heel lifts, and, in rare severe cases, walking casts for 2-4 weeks.

63-3. d. The middle third of the Achilles' tendon has a relatively avascular zone. It can develop so called areas of mucinoid degeneration due to excessive torque, twisting, repetitive microtrauma, or tears. Finally, aging of the tendon in some individuals can lead to these changes. This can leave the tendon susceptible to rupture with rapid eccentric loading. Management of acute ruptures usually requires surgical repair.

63-4. b. Heel pain syndrome results from excessive pull of the plantar fascia at its insertion on the calcaneus. Elevating the heel results in shortening of the arch, which relieves tension of the plantar fascia. Soft large long arch supports, almost like a rocker-bottom insert, are quite helpful as well. Negative heels would have the opposite effect.

63-5. b. The posterior tibial tendon in the closed kinetic chain assists in heel raise and inversion of the subtalar joint. Integrity of this muscle-tendon unit can be assessed by the single limb toe raise maneuver. Failure of the subtalar joint to resupinate and the heel to invert indicates posterior tibial tendon dysfunction.

CHAPTER **64**

Biomechanics of Running and Gait

Karl B. Fields, MD

Mitchell W. Craib, MA

Murray E. Allen, MD

QUESTIONS

64-1. Biomechanics describes external and internal forces that affect a biological system. Which of the following is *not* a true statement regarding these forces?
   a. translational movement places the least stress about joints of the lower extremity.
   b. examples of external forces include wind resistance, gravity, ground reaction, and friction.
   c. external impact forces for running range from two to four times body weight.
   d. internal impact forces for the ankle and knee are about half of external impact forces.
   e. the force peak for pushoff exceeds that for impact.

64-2. Running gait and walking gait differ. Which one of the following is *not* a true statement?
   a. both running and walking involve a swing and stance phase.
   b. stance phase in running is only one third as long as in walking.
   c. the float phase of walking is very brief, less than one fourth that of running.

d. some degree of compensatory pronation is present in rear foot motion during both running and walking.

e. pelvic rotation and adduction of the hip and thigh allow running to occur along a single vector, whereas walking occurs along two parallel vectors.

64-3. All of the following are true concerning eccentric muscle contraction, EXCEPT:

a. eccentric contractions pose a low risk of musculotendinous injury.

b. eccentric contractions stimulate the "stretch-shortening cycle" of muscle activity, which results in more powerful muscle action.

c. eccentric contraction of the hamstring helps stabilize the knee during initial foot strike.

d. eccentric implies that the muscle is lengthened while contracting.

e. running uphill may stimulate a more powerful eccentric contraction of the gastrocnemius.

64-4. Orthotics are *most* effective in a runner with:

a. leg length inequality.

b. plantar fasciitis.

c. metatarsalgia.

d. cavus feet.

e. excessive pronation.

64-5. The basic principle that underscores the use of prepared orthotic inserts for runners is that:

a. runners get too much impact to prevent breakdown in the lower extremity.

b. most runners have anatomical flaws that merit corrective therapy.

c. once a runner has been injured, permanent form changes occur that require orthotic correction.

d. without the preventive use of orthotics mileage >40 per week will ultimately lead to injury.

e. subtalar neutral is the best anatomical position for runners.

The following questions relate to some of the common running disorders known collectively as "shin splints." Each clinical entity will be highlighted with a patient's name, and questions about that case will be related to that patient's name.

CASE #1

Clinton (male aged 23) tells you (his doctor) that he had "shin splints" that had been increasing in severity over the last several months. He had run a few marathons before at a somewhat slow pace, and decided to concentrate on middle distances, where he thought he might be competitive. To pick up his speed, he had added some very intense sprint training to his regime. Lately, he found that part way through a distance training run his leg would hurt. He would be running with little discomfort when within about 30 seconds a deep dull pain occurred along the medial side of his lower leg about the middle half of this leg, and became so severe that it literally stopped him in the middle of a stride. He said he had a high pain threshold but could not run through this pain. About 2 minutes later the pain would mysteriously subside and so he could start running again, but within moments the pain would recur. He would have to walk home. The pain would build from a mild dull ache to severe anguish in 20 to 30 seconds. Later that night and the next day he would feel fine. At the time of examination, he had been off running for 3 days and specific points of leg tenderness could *not* be found on examination. (You have a clinical diagnosis on **Clinton's** case, which will be inferred by your management of this case.)

64-6. In **Clinton's** case, what single investigation would most likely give you a positive diagnosis?
  a. technetium 99m scan.
  b. oblique radiography.
  c. "slit catheter" analysis.
  d. computerized tomography (CT) scan.

64-7. In **Clinton's** case, presuming that the investigations confirmed your diagnosis, what would be your initial therapy?
  a. air cast.
  b. reduce sprint and distance training.
  c. diuretics.
  d. supplemental iron.
  e. corrective foot orthoses.

64-8. **Clinton** is a demanding competitive athlete, a rising star, but despite your best therapy (above plus more) he did not improve. What is your next treatment direction?
  a. short leg walking cast.
  b. surgical compartment release.
  c. parenteral iron.
  d. electromagnetic stimulation.
  e. ultrasound and laser modality therapy.

CASE #2

Hillary (female aged 19) started a running program 5 months ago to stay in shape. She also started a vegetarian diet but is not strict about it. She does aerobic exercises as well but has never run much before. She says she has "shin splints" and describes a pain in her lower leg that has been building in severity over the last month. She could initially run through the pain, which occurred part way through a run, but now lasts through the night and for the next several days. If she has not run for several days, her leg is still quite tender to touch. She is continuing her aerobic exercises at a reduced intensity and stopped running 2 weeks ago. Examination reveals not only a **very tender focal point** along the lower third tibial margin of the affected side, but also a lesser pain on the other leg, which was a surprise to her. She was observed to hyperpronate when she jumped and ran; otherwise, there were no obvious biomechanical abnormalities.

64-9. In **Hillary's** case what single investigation would most likely give you a positive diagnosis?
   a. technetium 99m scan.
   b. oblique radiogram.
   c. "slit catheter" analysis.
   d. CT scan.

64-10. In **Hillary's** case, presuming that the investigations confirmed your diagnosis, what would be your most likely initial therapy?
   a. air cast.
   b. supplemental calcium
   c. estrogen supplements, contraceptive pill.
   d. supplemental protein.
   e. corrective foot orthoses.

64-11. **Hillary** has been relatively inactive (no running or sports) for the last 4 weeks and is becoming quite impatient with your slow treatment. She says she has no more pain, but examination shows she is still tender in the lower third tibia. What is your next management approach?
   a. stop all physical activity; she should be using crutches to reduce weight bearing.
   b. introduce alternative "no stress" activity like swimming and upper body weight training.
   c. electromagnetic stimulation.
   d. check or recheck hemoglobin and perhaps serum iron and ferritin.
   e. radiography of sella turcica.

CASE #3

Washington was told by his football coach that he has "shin splints." He has a vague nonfocal pain in his lower leg, which bothers him during play, lingers for a few hours after, and is still tender for a few days when he stops all activity. It bothers him the first night after a hard game but not the second or third nights. The pain has been present for the last 3 months, but he can persist with play and training although at a lesser level than before. If he plays hard on one day, the next day he will be in much pain even if his level of activity is gentle. After 4 or 5 days off, he can return to fairly hard play, but only for 1 day. He says he's had shin splints on and off for years. He started some hard sprint training a few months ago. At the time of examination he has been inactive for only 5 days; the tenderness along the medial border of the tibia extends from the upper middle third to the lower third of the tibia, especially with resisted foot plantarflexion. He hyperpronates slightly, but this was corrected by the orthoses you prescribed on his previous visits; his shoes break down in a normal fashion without evidence of pronation stress at this time.

64-12. In **Washington's** case, what is your clinical diagnosis?
   a. deep muscle compartment syndrome.
   b. anterior compartment syndrome.
   c. periostitis/periostalgia.
   d. stress fracture of tibia.
   e. stress fracture of fibula.

64-13. For **Washington,** presuming that you confirmed your diagnosis, what would be your initial therapy?
   a. air cast.
   b. electromagnetic stimulation.
   c. steroid injections.
   d. transcutaneous electrical nerve stimulation.
   e. rest, ice packs, compression, elevation.

64-14. **Washington** is a rising star, but despite your best therapy he has not improved and insists on something that will either make or break his entry into professional football. What is next?
   a. long leg walking cast.
   b. electromagnetic therapy.
   c. surgical compartment release.
   d. surgically plate the tibia.
   e. fascial/periosteal release and debridement.

ANSWERS

64-1. c. Running places high levels of stress on joints of the lower extremity. This stress is lowest for pure translational movement and increases with torque. To run efficiently, runners must overcome a variety of external forces including wind, gravity, ground reaction, and surface friction. While external impact varies from two to four times body weight, depending on a variety of factors including running speed, internal impact forces to the lower extremity are much higher. Maximal active forces related to muscular activity are required for pushoff, and so force plates measure higher peaks during pushoff.

64-2. c. The gait cycle for both running and walking involves a stance and swing phase. The stance phase in running is brief, usually only one third that of walking. Running also involves a float phase not present in walking during which the individual has both feet airborne. Foot biomechanics are generally similar, with compensatory pronation allowing the foot to transfer weight from a supinated footstrike to a pronated foot for toeoff. The increased joint motion present in running allows runners to run more of a "straight line" along a single vector as opposed to walkers who progress along parallel vectors.

64-3. a. Eccentric contractions stimulate the initiation of the stretch-shortening cycle, which results in more powerful concentric contractions. Essentially, eccentric means that muscles lengthen while firing. A greater stretch such as occurs in running uphill may stimulate a more powerful eccentric contraction of muscles like the gastrocnemius. Since force is greatest during eccentric contractions, they logically pose a greater risk for musculotendinous injury and this has been confirmed by clinical observation.

64-4. e. In each of the clinical series that has been done for orthotics, clinicians noted improvement in a variety of conditions including leg length inequality, plantar fasciitis, and metatarsalgia. However, in each series runners with excessive pronation were the ones most likely to benefit from orthotics. Laboratory analysis has shown that the Achilles' tendon angle, which can be used as a measure for the degree of pronation, can be lessened by an orthotic with a medial wedge. Cavus feet carry the highest injury risk, but their response to orthotics is less predictable. Flexible, soft orthotics appear to work best in runners with cavus foot structure.

64-5. e. Fortunately, most runners do not have serious biomechanical or anatomical problems and can tolerate relatively high mileage and the impact of running without the use of special shoes or orthotics. However, runners who are not in a subtalar neutral position tend to have excessive pronation. Pronation appears clinically to be a factor in most of the major running injuries. For this reason orthotics were developed based on the principle that placing runners in a subtalar neutral position would lessen risk of injury.

64-6.   c. Clinton's case sounds like a muscle compartment problem. Think of muscles as fast turnover structures; as such, the onset and decline of symptoms can be very fast. Slit catheter systems can measure the muscle pressure and confirm the diagnosis.

64-7.   b. Relative rest is important, and instructing the runner not to provoke this problem is important; they should not try to run through this pain for fear of damaging the muscles. The other approaches to help shin splint pain do not work for muscle compartment disorders.

64-8.   b. In resistant cases, which are not uncommon in serious runners, surgery is required. The benefits can be quite dramatic, and some world class times have been recorded afterwards in athletes who would otherwise be doomed.

64-9.   a. Hillary has a stress fracture. Think of bones as being slow turnovers. The condition starts slow, but takes long to recover. The focal pain is a key. Radiography is helpful in about 25% of stress fracture cases. The bone scan is diagnostic; usually a very evident focal hot spot can be visualized.

64-10. e. None of these approaches are actually the best. The approach is to unload the tibia and give it unprovoked time to heal. Alternative sports help during the wait. Air casts, calcium, iron, estrogen, or protein have not been shown to help. Many athletes with stress fractures have them, in part due to excess foot pronation, which stresses the posterior tibialis muscle and soleus where they attach at the posterior lower third of the tibia, the common site of stress fractures in runners. Here the orthotics help, usually not right away but later on once they start running again. It might help to prevent stress fractures the second time around. Some athletes will feel a considerable relief to their shin splints right away with orthotic use, but this is not likely a change in the bone, but possibly a relief to stress of the above muscles.

64-11. b. Impatient athletes cannot be told to "stop"; they dislike negative instructions. Get them into something intense but not tibia loading. Implore them to take the opportunity to cross-train and learn another sport.

64-12. c. This is a cousin of tibia stress, but instead of the bone cracking, the overlying periosteum probably avulses along its attachment where the posterior tibialis and soleus pull. Think of the periosteum as intermediate between muscle and bone, and its clinical response is a little of both, like stress fractures and like muscle compartment problems. Periostitis (or periostalgia) can have focal points of pain, and also tender muscles. They appear to recover faster than stress fractures, but the relief of pain when they stop takes longer to be enjoyed than muscle compartment pain.

64-13. c. Local conservative therapy has not worked too well for this problem. Some clinicians have noted improvement with steroid injections. Usually, the best approach is time; unload the periosteum. This condition has a nasty habit of easily recurring.

64-14. e. Now the clinical situation is getting desperate. Conservative methods usually fail in periostalgia (not an "itis," there is not a lot of inflammation in this condition). Surgery is sometimes helpful and often will find quite a large buildup of granulation tissue along the periosteum, somewhat akin to repeated avulsion events at the periosteum.

C H A P T E R **65**

Ankle Taping and Bracing

Kirk Jones, MD

QUESTIONS

65-1. A patient presents with a recurring history of lateral ankle sprains. The most appropriate response would consist of the following:

a. casting followed by use of a bracing device for future sports participation.

b. besides the usual ice, compression, and elevation, no further action is necessary.

c. application of either ankle taping and/or bracing depending on the degree of swelling, followed by physical therapy for strengthening and proprioceptive gains.

d. the use of a prophylactic device in all activities of daily living until surgery becomes inevitable.

65-2. Taping has been found to be effective in reduction of ankle sprains by:

a. significantly retaining the amount of ankle motion restriction at least 2 hours postapplication.

b. enhancing proprioceptive responses in ankles with significant talar tilt.

c. underlying mechanism may not be clearly understood.

d. a and b.

e. b and c.

65-3. In recommending the use of a prophylactic knee brace (PKB), one should be knowledgeable of the fact that:
  a. the exact mechanism of injury is difficult to replicate in laboratory situations.
  b. research both supports and refutes injury reduction as the result of PKB use.
  c. cadavers make for easier reference of results to living subjects, therefore providing us with no controversy with regard to PKB use.
  d. a and c.
  e. a and b.

65-4. The American Academy of Orthopaedic Surgeons have classified knee braces by:
  a. their design of either hinged/post/strap or hinged/post/shell.
  b. their function of either derotational or detranslational.
  c. their function of either prophylactic, functional, or rehabilitative.

65-5. In deciding whether a functional knee brace (FKB) should be recommended to a patient with an anterior cruciate ligament–deficient knee, the following should be considered:
  a. FKBs are effective in eliminating knee subluxation.
  b. FKBs should not be a substitute for a rehabilitative program.
  c. FKBs provide subjective improvement in reduction of laxity.
  d. a and b.
  e. b and c.
  f. all of the above.

ANSWERS

65-1. c. Both ankle taping and/or bracing can be used postinjury, with taping the method of choice if reduction of swelling is desired. Initially, bracing can be used over a tape job and then can be used solely. A rehabilitative program should follow for prevention of further episodes by focusing on improvement of strength and proprioceptive training.

65-2. e. Taping has been reported to enhance proprioceptive responses in ankles with significant talar tilt. Taping does not provide major or prolonged stabilization for an ankle. Its mechanism for reducing ankle sprains in athletes without previous injury is not clear. Further research is required.

65-3. e. Recommendation for the use of a PKB is difficult due to the inability to test the mechanisms that lead to injury in the field and also due to the fact that research is controversial in determining whether PKBs have actually led to injury reduction in epidemiological studies. Cadaver use does not provide for dynamic stability or soft tissue compliance as found with in vivo situations.

65-4. c. Knee braces are classified according to the function they provide, namely, prophylactic, rehabilitative, and functional. These classifications are somewhat arbitrary, and some manufacturers make claims for their braces that include all categories.

65-5. e. FKBs have been found to subjectively reduce the number of subluxations experienced by the wearer. FKBs should be used in conjunction with a rehabilitative program to achieve the best outcome.

CHAPTER **66**

Musculoskeletal Injuries Unique to Growing Children and Adolescents

Angela D. Smith, MD

QUESTIONS

66-1. Compared with long bones of a young adult, the long bones of a child:
   a. absorb less energy before fracturing.
   b. are less porous.
   c. are more likely to fracture rather than bend.
   d. have thicker periosteum.

66-2. Relatively frequent sites of adolescent osteochondritis dissecans related to *overuse* include:
   a. capitellum.
   b. femoral head.
   c. proximal tibia.
   d. radial styloid.
   e. talus.

66-3. In the unconscious child injured in a diving accident, cervical spinal cord injury may be ruled out when:
   a. normal cervical spine radiographs are obtained.
   b. the child has full, active, painless range of motion of the cervical spine and limbs.
   c. the child is awake and has normal cervical spine radiographs.
   d. the child is awake and neurologically intact.

66-4. Despite anatomic reduction and satisfactory healing, some fractures have a high incidence of subsequent growth arrest and deformity. Which of the following fractures is *most likely* to cause clinically significant growth arrest, even with appropriate treatment?
   a. 10-year-old skater falls onto her outstretched hand, sustaining a torus fracture of the distal radius.
   b. 11-year-old baseball player jams his arm sliding into base, sustaining a supracondylar humerus fracture.
   c. 12-year-old cyclist falls from her bicycle, inverting her ankle and sustaining a minimally open Salter-Harris type 4 fracture of the medial malleolus.
   d. 13-year-old football player is clipped by an opponent, sustaining a Salter-Harris type 2 fracture of his distal femur.

66-5. A skeletally immature adolescent with grade I spondylolisthesis:
   a. is likely to be asymptomatic.
   b. is unlikely to have spondylolysis.
   c. requires treatment with a brace.
   d. should not be allowed to play football.

66-6. An 11-year-old gymnast hyperextends her knee on a twisting dismount, and the knee joint rapidly fills with fluid. She is *least* likely to have sustained a:
   a. dislocation of the patella.
   b. fracture of the tibial eminence.
   c. partial tear of the anterior cruciate ligament.
   d. tear of the lateral collateral ligament.

66-7. In Legg-Perthes disease one of the following descriptions is *not* correct:
   a. the disease is a cause of painful "knee-type" limp in an active child.
   b. the probable etiology is avascular necrosis of the head of the femur.
   c. the age and sex preference is around 8 years, male.
   d. with early treatment, prognosis is good.
   e. the most secure treatment is early hip replacement surgery.

One of the following muscles is associated with one of the conditions mentioned in the questions below. Match the muscle most closely involved with the injury.
   a. gastrocnemius.
   b. hamstrings.
   c. quadriceps.
   d. rectus femoris.
   e. sartorius.

66-8. Sever's disease, calcaneal apophysitis.

66-9. Osgood-Schlatter disease, tibial apophysitis.

66-10. Avulsion of the anterior superior iliac spine.

66-11. A very active 14-year-old jumper noted increased pain and **swelling** following athletic activity. He/she could not remember any acute injury, but described episodes of locking of the knee, relieved by "twisting it back and forth, and then straightening it with a popping sound." The likely diagnosis would include all EXCEPT:
   a. discoid lateral meniscus.
   b. grade I chondromalacia patella or patellofemoral pain syndrome.
   c. osteochondritis dissecans.
   d. parrot beak tear of medial meniscus.

66-12. In a young athlete who presents with symptoms and clinical findings of shoulder impingement, the most likely etiology is:
   a. entrapment/neuropathy of the long thoracic nerve to serratus anterior leading to instability.
   b. degenerative acromioclavicular (AC) joint or spurs on the underside of the acromion.
   c. inadequate dynamic stabilization of the shoulder (weak muscle) and/or glenohumeral instability.
   d. acromioclavicular joint capsulitis.

66-13. In the young baseball player who presents with an **insidious** onset of episodes compatible with locking of the elbow, the most likely etiology is:
   a. an inflammatory disorder of the elbow with impingement of the hypertrophied synovium.
   b. radial head fracture with residual loose body.
   c. tear of the ulnar collateral ligament.
   d. osteochondritis dissecans of the capitellum.

ANSWERS

66-1. d. The child's long bone, as compared to the adult's, has thicker periosteum, is more porous, and can absorb more energy in part through bending.

66-2. a. Osteochondritis dissecans (OCD) of the capitellum is a relatively frequent cause of elbow pain among pitchers and gymnasts. OCD of the femoral head in adolescents rarely occurs other than as a sequela of Legg-Perthes disease. OCD of the talus is more often related to an osteochondral injury than to repetitive microtrauma alone. To my knowledge, no case of OCD related to overuse of the proximal tibia or radial styloid in an adolescent has been reported.

66-3. d. A young child with a complete transection of the cervical spinal cord may have normal cervical spine radiographs on arrival at the hospital. Therefore, if there is any question of cervical spine trauma, the spine should be protected until the child is awake and has been found to have no neurological deficit. Remember that the head of a child is proportionately larger than an adult, so that immobilization on a standard spine board causes flexion of a child's cervical spine. Special children's spine immobilization boards are available, or a support can be placed under the shoulders to place the cervical spine in neutral alignment.

66-4. d. A torus, or buckle, fracture of the distal radius is generally a relatively low impact injury, with force absorbed by the metaphyseal bone. Enough compression injury to cause sufficient trauma to the physeal cells is apparently rare, and some question whether growth arrest ever occurs from pure compression of the distal radius. The supracondylar humerus fracture does not involve the growth plate. A typical 12-year-old girl has very little growth remaining in her ankle. Although physeal injury could occur even following anatomical reduction and fixation of an open type 4 fracture, it would be less likely to cause clinically significant growth abnormality than the distal femur fracture. Because the growth plate of the distal femur has an undulating architecture, much damage occurs to the physeal cells as the exposed growth plate of the fracture fragment (the distal piece) shears across remaining growth plate and the metaphyseal corner of the femur (the proximal piece). Therefore, even with anatomic reduction and fixation, growth abnormality is not unusual. The average 13-year-old boy has 3 cm of growth remaining in the distal femur, so significant angular deformity or even mild leg length discrepancy may occur. Therefore children who sustain these fractures must be monitored radiographically until it is clear that no clinically significant growth arrest is likely to occur.

66-5. a. It is unknown what proportion of the population who have mild spondylolisthesis are symptomatic. However, given the high incidence of spondylolisthesis and the relative infrequency of presentation of patients with spondylolisthesis and pain, most are presumably asymptomatic. One of the most frequent etiologies of spondylolisthesis in adolescence is spondylolysis. Only some symptomatic patients require brace treatment, and most spine surgeons allow skeletally immature adolescents with grade I spondylolisthesis to play football. Regular radiographic monitoring of the degree of slip is recommended.

66-6. d. Dislocation of the patella, fracture of the tibial eminence, and tear of the anterior cruciate ligament all frequently occur from the same mechanism—rotation of the femur medially relative to the fixed tibia, in nearly full extension. The rapidly developing hemarthrosis is caused by tear of the retinacular vessels and/or osteochondral fracture in dislocation of the patella, by bone bleeding in fracture of the tibial eminence, and by tearing of the ligament vessels (with or without additional vascular injuries such as peripheral tears of the menisci) in partial tear of the anterior cruciate ligament. Isolated lateral collateral ligament injuries are rare. Also, since the lateral collateral ligament is extraarticular, tears of this ligament do not cause rapid development of an intraarticular effusion.

66-7. e. In Legg-Perthes, all the first four answers are classic situations. The first line of treatment is conservative, to unload the hip for the femoral head to revascularize without collapse. In the widely abducted hip, the load is off the femoral head.

66-8. a. The gastrocnemius, part of the achilles tendon complex attaches to the calcaneus, where with respected tension strains can sometimes lead to an enthesopathy of the achilles-calcaneal attachment. This is called Sever's disease, a more anatomically, calcaneal apophysitis.

66-9. c. Osgood-Schlatter disease is an enthesopathy at the tibial tubercle due presumably to repetitive quadriceps pull via the patella and patellar tendon.

66-10. e. If the sartorius pulls hard enough, it can avulse its origin at the anterior superior iliac spine.

66-11. b. Meniscal and chondral disorders can be associated with pops and locking, but minor chondromalacia patella or patellofemoral pain is not.

66-12. c. The gangly young "skeletally immature" athlete often can be unstable in the shoulders and present as if impingement. It takes years for the skeleton to mature and handle the tasks that strong athletes handle easily, yet the young athlete often attempts to emulate his older heroes.

66-13. d. This is not an acute injury scenario but rather one of repetitive strain. Chondral injuries can occur under such circumstances. During the pitching motion, when the arm is accelerating forward from the cocked position, the capitellar chondral surface is exposed to compressive strain.

C H A P T E R **67**

Rehabilitation for Children and Adolescents

Angela D. Smith, MD

QUESTIONS

67-1. The earliest phases of a rehabilitation program for an avulsion fracture include all of the following, EXCEPT:
    a. determination of flexibility deficits.
    b. determination of short-term goals.
    c. proprioceptive training.
    d. range of motion exercises.

67-2. To best encourage a young athlete's compliance with a rehabilitation program:
    a. make it inclusive.
    b. make it short.
    c. make it very repetitive.
    d. make it very simple to do.

67-3. Of the rehabilitation exercises below, the most important exercise for treating a 14-year-old runner with patellofemoral pain is:
    a. hamstring curls.
    b. hip flexor stretches.
    c. straight leg raises.
    d. terminal arc flexions.

67-4. Weight-training programs for children may be unsafe if:
   a. flexibility exercises are included.
   b. machines are adjusted for height.
   c. repetitions number greater than 10.
   d. resistance is 1 maximum repetition.

67-5. Stretching exercises for a hockey team of 8 year olds should emphasize:
   a. gentle bouncing.
   b. partner stretching.
   c. performing each stretch five times.
   d. sustained stretching for 15-30 seconds.

ANSWERS

67-1. c. Avulsion fractures are often related to specific flexibility deficits. Although it is usually impossible to test the flexibility of the muscles attached to the avulsed region initially because of pain, it is important to check the same muscles on the opposite extremity as well as the other muscle groups. By doing this, the rehabilitation program can be designed to address these flexibility deficits early on. A critical component of the early rehabilitation program is to establish immediate and short-term goals of the program. Gentle range of motion exercises are started as soon as pain allows, but proprioceptive training of the injured region generally is begun only in the later phases of the rehabilitation program.

67-2. b. Young athletes tend to have a shorter attention span and even less patience with injury than adults. Therefore they are more likely to be compliant with a rehabilitation program that addresses the most important factors in their rapid, safe return to sport than with one that is all inclusive. It may be desirable to correct all of the athlete's deficits in strength, flexibility, endurance, proprioception, biomechanics, and cardiorespiratory fitness, but it is generally more practical to recommend a few exercises that are interesting and can be varied slightly or progressed rapidly to avoid the boredom of exercises that are too repetitive or too easy. If you can make it fun as well, so much the better.

67-3. c. The quadriceps, primarily the vastus medialis obliquus, usually require strengthening in young patients with patellofemoral pain. This can be done by straight leg raises, terminal arc extension exercises, or minisquats. Simple straight leg raise progressive resistance exercises with ankle weights have proved extremely effective in treating the type of patient discussed here. In these patients also look for leg malalignment factors that could exacerbate valgus knee strains, such as foot hyperpronation.

67-4. d. To avoid injury, children should concentrate on lifting submaximal weights multiple times, rather than the maximum that they can lift once. One repetition maximums can cause acute injuries.

67-5. d. Minimal additional lengthening of a muscle is obtained in the fourth and fifth bouts of stretching done in a single session. Therefore performing each stretch for 15-30 seconds two to three times is reasonable. Hockey athletes of this age rarely understand the concept of the safe, pulsed stretching that is often done by dancers, so they are best taught to perform sustained, gradual stretches. Encouraging stretching of a child by an untrained, vigorous teammate could easily lead to injury, so partner stretching is not appropriate in this setting.

CHAPTER **68**

Strength Training for Children and Adolescents

Sally S. Harris, MD, MPH

QUESTIONS

68-1. Children and adults show similar gains in strength after an appropriate program of strength training in terms of:
   a. absolute strength gains.
   b. relative strength gains (% improvement).
   c. both.
   d. neither.

68-2. All of the following are important mechanisms for strength gain as a result of strength training for preadolescents, EXCEPT:
   a. increases in muscle size (muscle hypertrophy).
   b. increased intrinsic contractile muscle function (twitch torque).
   c. improved motor skill coordination.
   d. increased neural drive.

68-3. Which one of the following statements is true?
   a. strength training during childhood places an individual at greater risk for musculoskeletal injury than participation in other sports and recreational activities.
   b. prepubertal children are more prone to strength training–related injury than older children or adults.

    c. strength training programs have detrimental effects on flexibility in children.

    d. all of the above statements are true.

    e. none of the above statements are true.

68-4. Prior to skeletal maturity (Tanner stage 5) it is recommended that children and adolescents avoid all of the following, EXCEPT:

    a. strength training involving several sets of multiple repetitions of submaximal resistance.

    b. Olympic-style lifts.

    c. power lifting.

    d. body building.

    e. all of the above.

68-5. Which of the following statements regarding strength training in children and adolescents is *not* true?

    a. the most common site of injury is the lower trunk.

    b. the most common type of injury is sprains and strains.

    c. the majority of injuries appear to be preventable by avoiding improper technique, excessive loading, ballistic movements, and lack of supervision.

    d. prepubescent children engaging in strength training have a significant risk of epiphyseal fracture.

68-6. Children and young adolescents should *not* be involved in weight training because:

    a. their tissues are too weak and thus exposed to easy injury.

    b. they are too young and lack the social maturity to learn the safety skills of weight training.

    c. there is no weight-training equipment suitable for their size.

    d. they are subject to "growth arrest" at the epiphysis with intense weight training.

    e. none of the above are true.

ANSWERS

68-1. b. Prepubescent children make similar relative strength gains compared to later stages of pubertal development and adulthood but demonstrate smaller absolute strength increases.

68-2. a. Strength training prior to adolescence has little if any effect on muscle size (hypertrophy); training-induced strength gains are largely independent of changes in muscle size. Neurological adaptations such as increased neural drive, increased intrinsic contractile muscle function, and improved motor skill coordination are more important mechanisms of strength gain for children.

68-3. e. There is no evidence that children involved in strength training are at increased risk of injury compared to adolescents or adults or to children that participate in other sports or recreational activities. There appear to be no detrimental effects on flexibility.

68-4. a. The competitive sports of weight lifting (Olympic lifting), power lifting, and body building, which typically involve lifts with maximal amounts of weight and/or ballistic maneuvers, are not recommended for children prior to skeletal maturity (Tanner stage 5) due to the potential for injury associated with extremely high loads or physical stress on the immature skeleton. High repetitions with low weights have been shown to be safe.

68-5. d. Epiphyseal fracture is a relatively rare occurrence in sports in general, and there is no evidence to suggest that strength training presents any greater risk in this regard than other sports and recreational activities. Prepubescents do not appear to be at increased risk, as the majority of these injuries have occurred in pubescents and adolescents (none in children less than age 12).

68-6. e. As with the theme of this set of questions, it would appear that past warnings to adolescents were meant to keep them out of the gym, where bad elements might lurk. Doctors may have at times been recruited to support such warnings.

C H A P T E R **69**

Fracture Diagnosis and Management of Common Injuries

Michael E. Robinson, MD

QUESTIONS

69-1. A 25-year-old man fell on his extended right hand 1 week ago while rollerblading. At physical examination he was found to have persistent wrist pain which was particularly tender in the snuffbox area. You think he may have a scaphoid fracture, and you order radiographs. No fracture is noted, but the anteroposterior film shows a widened scapholunate distance, which may indicate scapholunate dissociation (a clinically significant ligamentous injury). Which one of the following scapholunate angle measurements would be most helpful in confirming this diagnosis?
   a. 30 degrees.
   b. 45 degrees.
   c. 65 degrees.
   d. 80 degrees.

69-2. Which one of the following statements about field treatment of fractures is most correct?
   a. splinting of fractures in the field wastes valuable time, which could be used for transportation.
   b. splinting of fractures in the field facilitates transportation of the patient and obtaining radiographs.

    c. splinting with gentle longitudinal traction should not be attempted because of the risk of further soft tissue (especially neurovascular) damage.

    d. splinting should be performed only with approved devices such as an inflatable air splint.

69-3. In which of the following pediatric fractures could you expect residual bony angulation to correct spontaneously?

    a. moderate valgus angulation of a midshaft tibia fracture.

    b. moderate volar angulation of a fracture of the distal metaphysis of the radius.

    c. moderate varus angulation of a midshaft tibia fracture.

    d. moderate rotation of a distal humerus fracture.

69-4. Which of the following treatment protocols would be most appropriate for a nondisplaced radial head fracture without mechanical block?

    a. posterior elbow splint for 2 weeks with early range-of-motion exercises and increasing strengthening and functional activities as tolerated.

    b. long arm cast for 6 weeks followed by range-of-motion exercises and strengthening and functional activities.

    c. figure-8 brace for 4 weeks with early range-of-motion exercises and advancing strengthening and functional activities as tolerated.

    d. short arm thumb spica cast for 2 weeks followed by range-of-motion exercises and strengthening and functional activities.

69-5. Which one of the following statements most correctly describes the fracture pictured in Fig. 69-1?

    a. transverse distal radius fracture with 65 degrees of dorsal angulation.

    b. spiral distal radius fracture with complete volar displacement and 1-cm shortening.

    c. transverse distal radius fracture with complete dorsal displacement and 1-cm shortening.

    d. spiral distal radius fracture with 65-degree volar angulation.

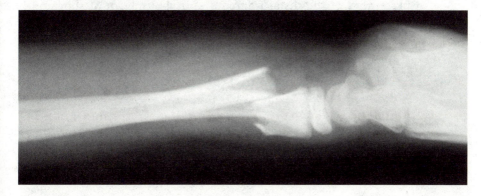

FIG. 69-1

ANSWERS

69-1. d. Scapholunate dissociation is the ligamentous analog of the scaphoid fracture. Because this condition is often treated surgically, the patient should be referred to a specialist. The mechanism of injury is a stress-loading fall onto the extended wrist, which results in localized edema and pain in the area of the anatomical snuffbox. A scapholunate gap of more than 4 mm on an anteroposterior radiograph is confirmatory, as is a scapholunate angle of 80 degrees on lateral radiographs. The normal scapholunate angle ranges from 30-60 ±15 degrees.

69-2. b. Splinting in the field provides pain relief and facilitates transportation of the patient and obtaining radiographs. Splinting the injury where it lies or with application of gentle longitudinal traction is acceptable. Any materials on hand may be used as an immobilizing device.

69-3. b. In children longitudinal growth from the epiphyseal plate helps correct some residual fracture angulation, especially if the fracture is close to the epiphysis and the angulation occurs in same plane of motion as the nearest joint. Varus and valgus angulation in the tibia occur at 90 degrees to the plane of motion of the knee and are unlikely to spontaneously correct. Rotational deformities also will not remodel. Mild to moderate volar or dorsal angulation of the radial metaphysis at the wrist can remodel with growth. In the long bones very accurate and well-aligned reductions are required.

69-4. a. Nondisplaced radial head fractures with no mechanical block to motion are appropriately treated with splinting for comfort and beginning early range-of-motion exercises as tolerated. Lengthy immobilization may actually impair functional recovery and increase disability. Figure-8 brace is used for clavicle fractures. Short-arm thumb spica cast is used for scaphoid fractures.

69-5. c. The x-ray shows a lateral view of a transverse distal radius fracture at the metaphyseal/diaphyseal junction with complete dorsal displacement of the distal fragment and about 1 cm of shortening. No angulation exists.

CHAPTER **70**

Overuse Injuries

Warren Scott, MD

QUESTIONS

70-1. Clinically medial tibial stress syndrome ("shin splints") refers to:
    a. periostitis of the tibia.
    b. myofasciitis of the medial compartment of the lower leg.
    c. stress fractures of the tibia.
    d. all of the above.

70-2. The final phase of the rehabilitation process is:
    a. strengthening all the injured muscle groups.
    b. stretching all the injured muscle groups.
    c. practicing proprioceptive exercises on an indoor balance board.
    d. practicing a sport-specific functional progressive skill that corresponds to your sport.

70-3. Overuse injuries in throwing sports such as tennis, volleyball, and baseball that occur at the shoulder:
    a. can be secondary to poor technique.
    b. can be related to excessive training to achieve a new skill.
    c. can become progressive and destructive to the myotendinous unit, such that surgical debridement may be necessary to heal the injury.
    d. all of the above.

261

70-4. A 40-year-old right-handed carpenter presents with a 6-month history of right elbow pain. He plays baseball (short stop) but doesn't remember any specific injury. Maybe, 6 months ago, he hyperextended it with a hard throw. The next day it was swollen and painful to bend for 2-3 weeks but seemed to get better. Now it aches when held in certain positions. It also seems to get sticky and wants to lock up. This occurs almost every day and interferes with his work. Past history includes elbow pain when he pitched Little League. The best approach to this patient is:

    a. radiograph of both elbows (anteroposterior, oblique, and lateral views).

    b. provide Ace wrap, ice, nonsteroidal antiinflammatory drugs, note to be off work, and stop baseball.

    c. refer to physical therapy for rehabilitation of the shoulder and elbow.

    d. after conducting a careful examination that confirms the patient's complaints, order a magnetic resonance imaging scan.

70-5. Most sports-related stress fractures:

    a. require rigid fiberglass immobilization for 6-8 weeks to allow full healing.

    b. require rigid fiberglass immobilization for 1-2 weeks and then flexible splints for 6-8 weeks to allow full healing.

    c. require prefabricated plastic braces with hinges to allow movement only in one plane at a time.

    d. require some type of protective support that allows movement but still protects against reinjury. Trial and error with a variety of braces and splints is the best approach. Protection may be necessary for many months.

ANSWERS

70-1. d. Shin splints is a common street term defining athletic lower leg pain. Pounding and twisting are the mechanism of injury. Adolescent growth, amenorrhea, and overload set up stress patterns that affect periosteum, bone, and muscle-tendon. Each athlete (and each sport) pounds and twists a little differently, thereby producing a variable injury pattern. Those athletes with various leg malalignment problems are more prone to shin splints.

70-2. d. All the above are useful in the rehabilitation process. Stretch and strengthen early in the rehabilitation process. Proprioceptive drills on balance boards precede game play. Sport-specific functional progressive skill building should be the final hurdle before return to competition.

70-3. d. Overuse is usually too much, too soon, too hard, too often. Applying new skills and equipment variations can be contributory. Training-stress-strain is in balance with adaptation and recovery. Achieving success requires a proper balance. Years of injury, healing, and reinjury can produce tissue damage and scar formation.

70-4. d. This patient provides a 6-month history of loose body in the elbow. The mechanical symptoms of sticking-locking produce pain and subsequent swelling. The history of pitcher's elbow as an adolescent is a risk factor. The inability to pinpoint the exact injury is expected. If the examination reveals locking and jamming, a loose body is usually the cause and should be removed. Many physicians would first identify the loose body on a magnetic resonance imaging or computerized tomography arthrogram, and occasionally it may be seen on a radiograph.

70-5. d. Most stress fractures do not require fiberglass casting. A variety of materials and techniques are available to aid athletes with specific sports-related problems. In general, the material should be lightweight, moldable, and easily attached. It should allow the fullest sports motion but still protect the injury site. As injury progresses from significant to mild, the braces can be modified to allow more movement and stress. Wearing a soft brace also serves to remind the athlete not to overuse the limb.

C H A P T E R **71**

Physiology of Musculoskeletal Growth

Mimi D. Johnson, MD

QUESTIONS

71-1. Which of the following statements is *not true?*
   a. The average age of peak height velocity in girls is 12.1 years.
   b. The pubertal growth spurt begins 2 years earlier in girls than in boys.
   c. The average age of peak height velocity in boys is 14.1 years.
   d. By menarche most girls have reached 65% of adult height.

71-2. Which of the following does not directly affect growing bone?
   a. mechanical stress.
   b. somatomedin C.
   c. sulfation factor.
   d. insulin.
   e. estrogen.

71-3. The distal femoral physis is more likely to be injured by a lateral blow to the knee during:
   a. Tanner stage I.
   b. Tanner stage II.
   c. Tanner stage III.
   d. Tanner stage V.

71-4. Which of the following statements is true?
   a. 80% of adult bone mass is formed during adolescence.
   b. Delayed menarche is not associated with decreased bone mineral density.
   c. Peak bone mineral density is attained by 15 years of age.
   d. Physical activity is associated with increased bone mineral density in both children and adolescents.

71-5. During the growth spurt an adolescent athlete may have an increased risk of developing all of the following, EXCEPT:
   a. rotator cuff tendinitis.
   b. iliac crest apophysitis.
   c. Osgood-Schlatter disease.
   d. apophyseal avulsion of the ischial tuberosity.

ANSWERS

71-1. d. Most girls have reached 90% to 95% of adult height by menarche, which occurs at a mean age of 12.7 years in American girls. The median height gain after menarche is 7.4 cm.

71-2. d. Intrinsic tension due to muscle force across the joints and repetitively applied external stresses can affect bone growth. Somatomedin C (production stimulated by growth hormone), sulfation factor, thyroxin, estrogen, and testosterone are involved in the physiological control of skeletal growth. Insulin does not directly influence growing bone.

71-3. c. During prepubescence (Tanner stages I and II) the physis and its attachment to the zone of Ranvier are stronger than the ligamentous structures around the joint. The opposite is true during midpubescence (Tanner stages III and IV). Epiphysiodesis occurs during Tanner stage V.

71-4. d. 50% of adult bone mass is formed during the second decade. Delayed menarche and secondary amenorrhea are associated with decreased bone mineral density in adolescents. Peak bone mineral density is usually attained by 20 years of age and starts increasing by 16 years of age.

71-5. a. During the growth spurt the combination of decreased flexibility of muscle groups, the presence of apophyses, and athletic activity places athletes at risk for developing overuse injuries such as traction apophysitis or acute injuries such as apophyseal avulsion. The growth spurt does not place them at risk for rotator cuff tendinitis, which is often associated with weakness of the rotator cuff and repetitive overhead activities.

CHAPTER 72

Finding and Correcting Flexibility Deficits for Injury Prevention and Rehabilitation

Angela D. Smith, MD

QUESTIONS

72-1. Which of the following structures *does not* cross two major joints?
   a. biceps femoris.
   b. iliotibial band.
   c. rectus femoris.
   d. tibialis posterior.
   e. triceps.

72-2. Athletes most prone to injury have the following characteristics:
   a. lax ligaments, weak muscles, inflexible muscles.
   b. lax ligaments, strong muscles, inflexible muscles.
   c. tight ligaments, weak muscles, inflexible muscles.
   d. tight ligaments, strong muscles, inflexible muscles.

72-3. Evidence that indicates that some injuries may be preventable includes work showing that:
   a. loose-jointed athletes have fewer injuries.
   b. more flexible quadriceps are related to anterior knee pain syndromes.
   c. resistance training strengthens connective tissue.
   d. stronger muscles absorb less energy before failure.

72-4. To best stretch the quadriceps, an athlete should stand with the knee flexed and the hip in:
   a. extension and abduction.
   b. extension and adduction.
   c. flexion and internal rotation.
   d. neutral flexion and external rotation.

72-5. The best way to test the flexibility of the hamstrings, minimizing confounding factors, is the:
   a. popliteal angle test.
   b. sit and reach test.
   c. standing toe touch test.
   d. straight leg raise test.

72-6. If you were limited to only one time in the day to stretch, the most important time to stretch to gain and retain flexibility for sport is:
   a. first thing in the morning.
   b. last thing at night before going to bed.
   c. before sports or practices.
   d. after sports or practices.
   e. during the game.

72-7. The length of time to hold a stretch to gain optimum (not maximum) flexibility benefit is:
   a. 1 to 3 seconds, as in a ballistic stretch.
   b. 10 seconds, repeated once.
   c. 60 seconds.
   d. 120 seconds.
   e. 5 minutes.

72-8. Pain and stiffness after resting and in the morning often suggest:
   a. joint inflammation.
   b. muscular strain.
   c. sleep apnea.
   d. psychological factors.
   e. cancer.

ANSWERS

72-1. d. Biceps femoris, iliotibial band, and rectus femoris cross both the hip and knee, triceps crosses the shoulder and elbow, but the tibialis posterior crosses only the ankle, if it is considered as a single joint complex.

72-2. a. The weak, tight but gangly jointed athlete is quite prone to injury.

72-3. c. The profile of the young athlete most prone to injury has been shown to include loose (hypermobile) joints, inflexible muscles, and weak muscles. Other work indicates that stronger muscles absorb more energy before failing. An inverse relationship has been found between quadriceps muscle flexibility and incidence of anterior knee pain syndromes among elite figure skaters. From the perspective of this question, only c relates to "prevention."

72-4. b. The rectus femoris is the quadriceps muscle that crosses both the hip and the knee and is therefore more likely to be inflexible than the remaining quadriceps muscles, since it is less frequently brought through a full range of motion during the usual activities of daily living and of most sports. To stretch the rectus femoris the most, the hip should be extended, the knee fully flexed, and the hip adducted. Internal rotation of the hip may then further increase the stretch slightly. This is a tricky stretch. Stand up and try it; when you add the internal rotation and adduction, you should feel the extra tension in your quadriceps.

72-5. a. The sit and reach test and the standing toe touch test (both the same principle) allow an individual with a higher trunk/arm:lower extremity ratio to appear to be more flexible than one with shorter trunk and arm length and longer legs, even though the hamstrings in the first individual may actually have less true flexibility. As a child grows, the body proportions change, leading to apparent (but not necessarily real) changes in flexibility by this test. The straight leg raise is not as reproducible as the popliteal angle test in many examiners' hands, since the popliteal angle test seems to catch the hamstrings on the prominence of the ischial tuberosity reliably. When performing the straight leg raise test, often a point of resistance is felt; then the muscle feels as if it slips off the prominence, and greater raising of the leg is immediately possible, even though the flexibility has not changed.

72-6. d. During physical activity and sports the muscles are used and will stay tight from their last position, which is usually in contraction. Stretching after activity will bring the muscle back out to its full length and will improve flexibility; although stretching before a game may be helpful for the game, it does not lead to overall increased flexibility.

72-7. b. This is quite controversial, but consensus is aiming at somewhere between 10 and 30 seconds. Long stretches tend to be boring, and compliance is low. Short stretches do not allow enough time for the series elastic component of muscle to reach length. The 10-second repeated stretch will not reach maximum, but it is a reasonable optimizing compromise.

72-8. a. Prolonged rest, such as sleeping overnight, can stiffen muscles but will aggravate an inflamed joint even more. Muscular strains hurt with use, not rest, even though activity or stretching of such strained muscles is a first-line treatment.

CHAPTER 73

Epidemiology of Injuries

James G. Garrick, MD

QUESTIONS

73-1. You are reading a report of a study of injuries in high school football players. Which of the following findings would lead you to believe that many of the injuries that actually occurred were not included in the report?
   a. 15% of the injuries were contusions and abrasions.
   b. 25% of the injuries were fractures.
   c. 30% of the injuries were sprains.
   d. 25% of the injuries were strains.

73-2. Epidemiological studies in sports medicine have resulted in significant contributions concerning injury prevention in all but which of the following circumstances?
   a. catastrophic neck injuries in football.
   b. sliding injuries in softball.
   c. cleat size/configuration and ankle injuries in football.
   d. stretching programs and musculotendinous injuries (strains) in track and field.

73-3. A "descriptive" study enumerating the injuries seen by a physician covering a state high school wrestling championship would:
   a. assist in predicting staffing and equipment needs for next year's championship.

b. allow documentation of the dangers of "weight cutting."

c. confirm that older wrestlers have higher injury rates than younger wrestlers.

d. predict the type of injuries you would expect to see during the season while serving as the team physician for a high school wrestling team.

73-4. You have been the team physician for a large high school football team for the past 5 years. Last year you observed that there was a twofold increase in hamstring strains. During the summer you have the coaches institute a conditioning program during which half of the team practices hamstring stretching and half concentrates on hamstring strengthening. The following season you observe that hamstring injuries are halved (compared to the previous year) in both groups. You can conclude:

a. that the frequency of occurrence of hamstring strains is related to conditioning.

b. that your stretching and strengthening program prevented injuries.

c. that stretching and strengthening programs are equally effective in preventing hamstring strains.

d. none of the above.

73-5. You want to establish the prevalence of patellar tendinitis in high school basket players. Your best source of information would be:

a. medical insurance claims.

b. records of training room visits by participants in a large, invitational tournament.

c. team records documenting the causes for missed practices during the season.

d. personal interviews with all team members.

ANSWERS

73-1. a. If all you read are the contusions and abrasions in a football team, something is missing.

73-2. d. Neck injuries, softball sliding, and cleats have been well studied, but the track and field stretching programs have not been researched well, and some controversy still exists.

73-3. d. Keep it simple and don't generalize your work. Descriptive work can spot some staffing and equipment needs but will miss some matters that you'll have to use some imagination to predict and won't show up in all years of study. Weight cutting has not been associated with high injury rates and would not likely show up in a descriptive study anyway since the athletes would not likely admit to it. Younger wrestlers have a higher rate of injury than the more mature experienced ones.

73-4. d. Again, don't overestimate the brilliance of your work. There may be other factors beyond stretching or strengthening that caused the injury rise in the first place and other unknown variables that reduced it the second season.

73-5. d. Patellar tendinitis can be easily missed or not reported. The only way of determining its incidence is to examine the athletes personally. Record keeping by others is quite unreliable for research purposes.

C H A P T E R **74**

Injuries in Football and Soccer

James M. Moriarity, MD

QUESTIONS

74-1. According to NCAA statistics, the sport with the highest injury rate is:
   a. spring football.
   b. fall football.
   c. women's soccer.
   d. men's soccer.

74-2. Prophylactic ankle bracing is most likely to benefit:
   a. all ankles.
   b. previously injured ankles.
   c. neither.
   d. both.

74-3. An athlete with mild head injury without loss of consciousness sustained during competition may:
   a. return to competition if the athlete demonstrates no loss of neurological function, has no symptoms at rest or with exercise provocation, and has been observed on the sidelines for at least 20 minutes.
   b. should always be withheld from the remainder of the game.
   c. should be reexamined after the competition is concluded.
   d. should not be permitted to practice for 1 week.
   e. a and c.

74-4. An athlete is struck on the left shoulder and experiences a burning sensation in his left arm and hand. Examination on the sideline indicates weakness of abduction and external rotation of his left shoulder and weakness of arm flexion. The most likely diagnosis is:
   a. shoulder subluxation.
   b. brachial plexus injury involving the C7 nerve root.
   c. brachial plexus injury involving the C5 nerve root.
   d. neck injury suggestive of spinal stenoses.

74-5. Which of the following muscles does *not* span two joints?
   a. rectus femoris.
   b. adductor longus.
   c. vastus medialis.
   d. biceps femoris.
   e. b and c.

74-6. During the game a key football player seeks your advice for a big bruise on his mid humerus, an area he has bruised before. He wants your quick solution and then to return to play. You suspect a sizable hematoma deep in the muscle. What is your initial approach?
   a. send him back onto the field; it will heal regardless of what you do.
   b. aspirate the hematoma, add a compressive bandage, then return him to play.
   c. aspirate the hematoma, add a compressive bandage, no play today, but OK in 1 to 2 days.
   d. rest in sling, arm flexed to stretch the offended muscle, light compressive bandage, ice frequently for 2 days, no arm activity or return to play until the swelling is resolved.
   e. rest, compression, ice, elevation, and no play for 2 months.

74-7. What disorder are you trying to prevent with the above protocol?
   a. disseminating hemolysis.
   b. myositis ossificans.
   c. chondritis dissecans.
   d. bacterial myositis.
   e. delayed onset overuse myositis.

ANSWERS

74-1. a. Spring football has the highest injury rate of all NCAA sports. Interestingly, both men's and women's soccer have a higher incidence of injury than fall football.

74-2. b. In a study of South African soccer athletes, prophylactic ankle bracing was found to reduce the incidence of recurrent injury (i.e., in ankles with previous sprains). No ability to prevent ankle injury in a previously uninjured ankle was found.

74-3. e. An athlete with mild head injury and no loss of consciousness may return to competition if the neurological examination is normal, the athlete is asymptomatic at rest and with exercise, and if a period of observation has elapsed. Often, athletes appearing normal following mild head trauma will develop progressive symptoms of memory loss, confusion, or headache over a period of 20-30 minutes. Athletes with symptoms of retrograde and especially antegrade memory loss, headache, disorientation, or confusion should not return to competition that day. All athletes with head injury should be reexamined before clearance for further practice is granted; they should be totally symptom-free, including headache.

74-4. c. Brachial plexus injuries are common in contact sports. They may be caused by nerve root impingement, stretch of the plexus, or direct trauma to the plexus. Weakness of abduction and external rotation of the shoulder and weakness of arm flexion indicate involvement of the deltoid, infraspinatus, and biceps in a distribution consistent with a C5-C6 injury.

74-5. e. The adductor longus and vastus medialis do not span two joints; the rectus femoris and biceps femoris do. The rectus femoris muscle acts as a knee extender and a hip flexor. The biceps femoris acts as a knee flexor and hip extender. To adequately stretch a muscle that spans two joints, both joints must be locked. Interestingly, the biceps femoris muscle has two components, the short head and the long head, and each is innervated by different nerves.

74-6. d. Note in this question that the right answer is the one that is longest and best describes a treatment. This athlete's hematoma should be treated by essentially wringing it out, with muscle stretch. If it was in the anterior thigh, you would try to flex the knee to maximum to put the muscle under tension. The light compression and ice are also helpful in reducing inflammation.

74-7. b. Hematomas that are undertreated, allowed to organize, and then retraumatized, will sometimes calcify.

CHAPTER **75**

Track and Field

Carol Otis, MD

Murray E. Allen, MD

QUESTIONS

75-1. Historically, track and field events were developed in response to:
   a. A need to develop strengths and skills for daily survival against a harsh environment.
   b. An outgrowth of training for solidiers.
   c. The need to develop group co-operation for wars against other tribes.
   d. The natural pruning rituals aimed at gaining the ardor of women.
   e. Political stratagems aimed at sorting power within a group.

75-2. Which sport has the LEAST danger for spectators and others:
   a. Shot put.
   b. Discus.
   c. Javelin.
   d. Hammer.
   e. Hurdles.

75-3. Which of the following jumping sports has the highest risk of serious injury:
   a. Pole vault.
   b. High jump.
   c. Broad jump.

d. Triple jump.

e. Hurdles.

75-4. Among the sprinting events, which ACUTE injury will most commonly side-line an elite athlete:

a. Achilles tendonitis.

b. Cardiac arrhythmia due to hypertrophic cardiomyopathy.

c. Shoe interface problems like turf toe or blisters.

d. Ankle sprains.

e. Hamstring/quadriceps strain-tear.

75-5. Among the distance events, which CHRONIC disorder is most likely to side-line an elite athlete:

a. Achilles tendonitis.

b. Shoe interface problems like turf toe or blisters.

c. Patello femoral pain syndrome.

d. Shin splints or stress fractures.

e. Hamstring/quadriceps strain-tear.

ANSWERS

75-1. b. Early Greek history suggests that the track and field movement was developed as an outgrowth of soldier training. All the other options would be tertiary benefits of being successful at sports, such as surviving a harsh environment, war games organization, politics, and women; some of these would be considered somewhat fickle.

75-2. c. The throwing sports can harm spectators and other athletes, such as errant shot puts, discus, javelin, or hammer. These can strike other persons with sometimes fatal outcomes. The hurdles pose little threat to others.

75-3. a. Among the jumping sports, the pole vault has the most risk. This is due to the demands for great strength, speed, timing, balance, and technical difficulty. The margins of error are slim, and the consequences can be grave. All the other sports have their own profile of risks, but the pole vault is the riskiest.

75-4. c. The ham-quad strain-tear is the commonest acute unjury in sprinters. Achilles tendonitis is common among runners, but it is a chronic repetitive strain disorder, not acute.

75-5. a. Achilles tendonitis is the chronic disorder most hazardous among distance runners. Shin splints and knee pains are less common among the elite athletes, in part due to the selection process over time, and that these disorders can be more readily treated than can achilles tendonitis.

C H A P T E R **76**

Basketball Injuries

Michael D. Jackson, MD

James L. Moeller, MD

David O. Hough, MD

76-1. Lateral anterior ankle impingement will commonly respond to which of the following treatment options?
a. proprioceptive ankle training.
b. ankle range of motion exercises.
c. stabilization of lateral ankle ligamentous instability.
d. nonsteroidal antiinflammatories (NSAIDs).

76-2. Semimembranosus tendinitis may mimic which of the following pathological conditions?
a. Baker's cyst.
b. pes anserine bursitis.
c. medial meniscal tear.
d. anterior cruciate ligament tear.

76-3. A 22-year-old basketball player presents with a history of wrist pain after falling and landing on his hand earlier the same day. On examination he has tenderness over the anatomical snuff box and pain with wrist dorsiflexion. Radiographs of the wrist are negative. Treatment plans may include all of the following, EXCEPT:
a. cock-up wrist splint.
b. repeat radiography in 2 weeks.

c. bone scan.

d. thumb spica cast.

76-4. A 15-year-old presents with a history of being "poked in the eye" during a basketball game the previous night. She complains of eye pain, increased tearing, and a feeling "like there's a grain of sand in my eye." The patient usually wears contact lenses but came in today wearing her glasses. A small corneal defect is noted after fluorescein staining. Treatment would include all of the following, EXCEPT:

a. continue to wear glasses only.

b. antibiotic drops or ointment four to six times daily.

c. eye patch.

d. daily follow-up until the lesion heals.

ANSWERS

76-1. c. Anterior ankle impingement is often the result of lateral ankle ligamentous instability. Therefore this pathological condition will benefit from stabilization of the ligamentous laxity. Proprioceptive ankle training, referred to as PNF, plays an important part in the rehabilitation of ankle sprains by helping reduce recurrence. Ankle range of motion exercises may increase symptoms in anterior ankle impingement, as increased dorsiflexion is typically painful to the athlete. NSAIDs may be of minor benefit, but the major pathology is osteophyte formation and its resultant impingement with forced dorsiflexion of the ankle that is not amenable to medications. Additional treatment options include heel elevation, use of a negative heel, or surgical removal of the osteophytes. In some cases, scarring of a small meniscus between the lateral fibula and the talus may respond to injections.

76-2. c. Semimembranous tendinitis commonly presents as vague medial knee pain and can mimic medial meniscal tear. Baker's cyst is a cystic swelling located in the popliteal fossa that presents as discomfort on full flexion or extension of the knee and in some cases can communicate with the semimembrane bursa. Pes anserine is composed of the conjoined tendons of the sartorius, gracilis, and semitendinosus muscles. Anserine bursitis presents as pain and tenderness over the medial aspect of the knee approximately 2 inches below the joint line and can be confused with semimembranosus tendinitis if not examined carefully. Anterior cruciate ligament tears may present with posterior knee pain but the primary findings are knee effusion and anterior laxity.

76-3. a. The question should raise suspicion of scaphoid fracture. Scaphoid fractures often do not reveal themselves on initial radiographs, and if this is the case, the patient should be placed in a thumb spica cast and repeat radiographs should be performed in 2 weeks. If there is a need for more prompt diagnosis, a bone scan should be ordered. A cock-up wrist splint does not provide adequate immobilization in a case of acute scaphoid fracture and should not take the place of a thumb spica cast.

76-4. c. In the case of a small corneal abrasion in a contact lens wearer, treatment includes antibiotic drops or ointment, cycloplegics may be used, and the contact lenses are to remain out until the eye is fully healed. An eye patch is not used (pressure eye patches are used in individuals who do not wear contact lenses whose abrasions are considered at low risk for infection). Follow-up should be daily until healing of the corneal epithelium has occurred. Antibiotics should then be used for an additional 1-2 days. Contact lens use may resume after treatment is complete and the eye feels perfectly normal for 3-4 days.

CHAPTER 77

Bicycling Injuries

Robert L. Kronisch, MD

QUESTIONS

77-1. The correct height of a bicycle saddle is one that places the knee:
   a. in full extension.
   b. in 5-10 degrees of maximum extension.
   c. in 15-20 degrees of maximum extension.
   d. in 25-30 degrees of maximum extension.
   e. in 45 degrees of maximum extension.

77-2. Traumatic injuries in bicyclists occur most frequently in the following order:
   a. upper extremity > lower extremity > head and face > trunk.
   b. upper extremity > lower extremity > trunk > head and face.
   c. upper extremity > head and face > lower extremity > trunk.
   d. lower extremity > upper extremity > trunk > head and face.
   e. lower extremity > head and face > upper extremity > trunk.

77-3. A cyclist comes to your office complaining of knee pain, and you diagnose patellar tendinitis. You would most likely:
   a. raise the saddle and advise the cyclist to use the large chainring more often.
   b. raise the saddle and adjust the cyclist's cleats.
   c. lower the saddle and move it forward slightly.

    d. advise the cyclist to switch to a fixed clipless pedal.

    e. accommodate a varus alignment with a lift placed between the pedal and the cyclist's shoe.

77-4. A cyclist comes to your office complaining of paresthesias of the hand in an ulnar nerve distribution associated with bicycling. You would consider all of the following, EXCEPT:

    a. ensure that the bicycle frame was the right size and advise the cyclist to possibly switch to a shorter handlebar stem.

    b. order nerve conduction studies and advise the cyclist to discontinue all cycling until symptoms resolve.

    c. advise the cyclist to get padded gloves and handlebar grips and change hand position less often while riding.

    d. raise the stem and consider switching to a different handlebar to get more upright.

77-5. A cyclist comes to your office complaining of neck pain, and on examination you find tender trigger points in the trapezius and levator scapulae muscles. There is no history of previous neck problems, and the examination findings are otherwise normal. In addition to treating the muscle spasms, you would advise the cyclist to:

    a. raise the handlebars slightly.

    b. change to a longer stem and move the saddle back slightly.

    c. ride with the elbows fully extended.

    d. get narrower tires.

ANSWERS

77-1. d. Saddle height is one of the most important aspects of correct bicycle fit. If the saddle is too low, excess knee flexion can lead to patellar or quadriceps tendinitis or patellofemoral pain. If it is too high, it can predispose the cyclist to hamstring tendinitis or iliotibial band friction syndrome. Correct saddle height is determined by measuring the angle of the knee from greater trochanter to lateral femoral condyle to lateral malleolus with the foot on the pedal at bottom dead center (6:00 position). This angle should be 25-30 degrees for most cyclists. Saddle fore and aft position may also have an influence on the angle of the knee and the biomechanics of the lower extremity while cycling. Correct saddle fore and aft position places the front of the patella directly over the axle of the front pedal when the feet are on the pedals in the 3:00 and 9:00 positions. Adjustment of saddle height and/or fore and aft position may be indicated if any of the above conditions are diagnosed.

77-2. c. Traumatic injuries in bicyclists are much more common in the upper body than the lower body. Most injuries are superficial and minor in nature. The upper extremity is usually injured while trying to break a fall, which may lead to fractures of the scaphoid, distal radius, or the radial head or neck. Facial injuries are common and may be associated with underlying head injury. Concussions are relatively common, particularly in off-road bicycling, even with proper helmet use. Off-road cyclists are often thrown from their bicycles, which may increase the severity of injury. Severe or fatal bicycle injuries usually involve a collision with a motor vehicle. Fractures of the lower extremity and injuries to the abdomen and chest (other than rib fractures) are uncommon in cyclists.

77-3. b. Anterior knee complaints comprise the largest group of lower extremity overuse injuries seen in cyclists. In most cases there is an underlying training error, anatomical variant, or error in bicycle fit. Common training errors are overuse of the large chainring, training increases without an adequate training base, and sudden increases in mileage, intensity, or hill training. Anatomical variants such as patellofemoral malalignment, tibial rotation, overpronation, and valgus or varus alignment can place abnormal loads on muscles, joints, and tendons and may lead to inflammation and pain. These variations must be accommodated with adjustments to the bicycle. The saddle may need to be raised or moved back slightly to decrease the amount of knee flexion. The cyclist's cleats may need to be adjusted to better reflect the alignment of the lower extremities. A fixed clipless pedal does not allow any rotation of the foot while pedaling and may need to be switched to a floating clipless pedal. Some of the newer clip pedals allow more waffeling. Valgus alignments are accommodated with lifts or shims placed between the pedal and the shoe or with anterior wedged orthotics. Varus alignments are accommodated with spacers placed between the crankarm and the pedal.

77-4. b. Ulnar nerve compression at Guyon's canal is the most common overuse syndrome of the upper extremity associated with bicycling. The superficial location of the ulnar nerve at the wrist predisposes it to external compression, and the position of the hands on the handlebar combined with the shock and vibration transmitted from the riding surface are often etiological factors. Conservative treatment is almost always effective. This includes relative or complete rest with avoidance of pressure to the ulnar palmar area until symptoms resolve, which may take up to 3-6 months. Nerve conduction studies are rarely needed. Padded gloves and grips may help decrease the shock transmitted to the cyclist, and frequent changing of hand position on the handlebars may decrease compression of the nerve. The cyclist's reach should be adjusted so that no more than one-third of the body's weight is placed on the handlebars. This usually involves raising or shortening the handlebar stem. Occasionally it may be necessary to switch to a different type of handlebar that places the cyclist's upper body in a more upright position. Off-road cyclists should consider adding a front suspension system to their bicycle, or adjusting it if one is already present.

77-5. a. Neck pain is a common problem among cyclists. It is usually due to prolonged neck extension while cycling combined with shock and vibration transmitted to the cyclist from the riding surface. For cyclists who wear glasses they can easily slip down the nose, requiring more neck extension to see. Trigger points are more commonly found in the muscles on the left side of the neck, presumably from repeatedly turning the head to the left to look for backcoming traffic. In addition to the usual forms of treatment, cyclists often benefit from adjustments to the bicycle that decrease the amount of neck extension, get them more upright, and decrease the amount of shock and vibration transmitted to the neck area. Neck extension may be reduced by raising the handlebars or by shortening the cyclist's reach, which can be accomplished by moving the saddle forward slightly or by switching to a shorter handlebar stem. Shock and vibration to the neck area can be reduced by allowing the elbows to flex while riding, using padded gloves and handlebar grips, changing to a wider tire and/or lower inflation pressure, or by adding a front suspension system to the bicycle. Full range neck-specific exercises help to get the kinks out after a ride.

CHAPTER **78**

Running

Karl B. Fields, MD

QUESTIONS

78-1. In prospective trials of running injury, which two factors have the strongest association with running injury?
1. leg length inequality
2. running mileage >40 per week
3. excessive shoewear
4. previous injury
5. posterior tibialis muscle weakness
   a. 1 and 3.
   b. 1 and 5.
   c. 2 and 4.
   d. 3 and 5.
   e. 2 and 5.

78-2. A runner complains of persistent medial arch pain but has a rather unremarkable examination and a normal plain film of the foot. The logical next step in your management of this case is:
a. antipronation arch pad and reduction of training mileage by 50%.
b. bone scan or computerized tomography of the foot.

    c. physical therapy to emphasize ultrasound of the medial arch and posterior tibialis strengthening.

    d. ice massage, arch-strengthening exercise, and orthotics.

78-3. A runner complains of lateral knee pain and you suspect iliotibial band (ITB) syndrome. Ober's test is positive. This indicates that:

    a. bursal inflammation is present under the ITB.

    b. the lateral meniscus is also injured.

    c. the vastus lateralis is weak.

    d. the ITB is tight.

78-4. A runner has had chronic Achilles' problems and comes to see you because he has developed a dime-sized nodule over the Achilles tendon. All of the following are true, EXCEPT:

    a. injection of corticosteroid to the nodule with care to avoid the tendon substance will usually speed resolution.

    b. nodules may represent a partial rupture of the tendon.

    c. reduction in hill running and speed workouts will be key training changes during the recovery phase.

    d. heel lifts may reduce symptoms.

    e. ice massage reduces swelling.

78-5. For a runner with symptoms of patellofemoral stress syndrome (PFSS), which of the following would *not* fit the typical presentation?

    a. puffiness around the patella.

    b. increased Q angle.

    c. medial patellar tracking.

    d. vestus medialis obliquus (VMO) weakness.

    e. pronated gait.

ANSWERS

78-1. c. While leg length inequality, shoewear, and posterior tibialis muscle weakness have all been postulated among the multiple factors related to running injury, both mileage >40 per week and previous injury had a strong prospective association with running injury in the Ontario Cohort study.

78-2. b. While any of the listed treatments might have a role in certain conditions that cause pain over the medial arch, until navicular stress fracture is excluded as a diagnostic possibility, any of these approaches could cause further harm or delay proper treatment. Navicular fractures are quite resistant to conservative treatment; surgery is often required.

78-3. d. Ober's test helps indicate tightness of the ITB by failure of an unsupported lower extremity to drop with the force of gravity. The lateral meniscus and vastus lateralis are in no way tested by this maneuver. Inflammation is better demonstrated by knee flexion with or without varus stress.

78-4. a. Achilles' nodules must be assumed to be partial tears of the Achilles' with a "roll-up" of the tendon substance until proven otherwise. Corticosteroid may increase risk of rupture in weight-bearing tendons, and this approach carries risk. Other standard measures of Achilles' treatment may help speed resolution.

78-5. c. PFSS is the most common running injury and often presents in runners who have large Q angles and excessive pronation on running gait. Some of these individuals will have a true "miserable malalignment syndrome." Puffiness and even a small effusion are sometimes seen on inspection of the knee. VMO weakness is common, and most patients have some atrophy. This leads to abnormal patellar tracking with a tendency for the patella to track *laterally,* not medially.

CHAPTER **79**

Aquatic Sports

Lauren M. Simon, MD, MPH

QUESTIONS

79-1. A 14-year-old female swimmer complains of medial knee pain, which began after she increased her breaststroke yardage. She denies any previous knee injury, locking, swelling, or giving way. Which of the following structures is the most likely cause of her pain?
   a. medial collateral ligament.
   b. posterior cruciate ligament.
   c. lateral meniscus.
   d. anterior cruciate ligament.
   e. iliotibial band.

79-2. A mother brings her child with Down syndrome to your office requesting athletic clearance for him to participate in swimming. The child has been in good health and you identify no additional problems on his history and physical examination. Which of the following choices are correct?
   a. sign the preparticipation clearance form.
   b. obtain cervical spine radiographs.
   c. perform pulmonary function testing.
   d. perform exercise treadmill test.
   e. recommend gymnastics participation instead of swimming.

79-3. Which of the following is the most common cause of foot and ankle pain in swimmers?
a. athlete's foot.
b. anterior talofibular ligament sprain.
c. Morton's neuroma.
d. extensor tendinitis.
e. tarsal navicular stress fracture.

79-4. Apprehension shoulder is *most* likely to occur with which of the following strokes?
a. butterfly.
b. free-style.
c. breaststroke.
d. "head up" free-style.
e. backstroke.

79-5. A 14-year-old competitive diver complains of pain and slightly diminished hearing in her right ear for the past week. She denies any trauma to her ear. On examination you note an inflamed and tender right ear canal with some green discharge. *After* treatment, which of the following do you recommend to help prevent a recurrence of this problem?
a. clean ears daily with cotton swabs.
b. wear hard rubber ear plugs during diving practice.
c. instill a drying agent in the ears at the end of practice.
d. instill antibiotic otic drops in the ears for the entire season.
e. wear cotton in the ears for diving practice.

ANSWERS

79-1. a. The most common site of knee pain in swimmers, often breast-strokers, is the medial joint line or medial patellofemoral region. The breaststroker's knee pain has been correlated with increased age of the swimmer and increased breaststroke training distance, which can subject the knee to extreme valgus force during breaststroke kicks. The anterior cruciate ligament, posterior cruciate ligament, lateral meniscus, and iliotibial band are not considered sources of breaststroker's knee pain. The medial collateral ligaments are a reasonable candidate for the offended tissues.

79-2. b. Before clearing a child with Down syndrome to participate in swimming it is important to rule out atlantoaxial instability (AAI). There is a 15% incidence of AAI in children with Down syndrome; lateral cervical spine radiographs in neutral, flexion, and extension will identify most AAI. There is no indication to perform pulmonary function testing or exercise treadmill testing on this patient. People with AAI should avoid sports with risk for head and neck injury such as gymnastics, diving, and butterfly, breaststroke, and diving starts in swimming.

79-3. d. The repeated plantar flexion to neutral movements in dolphin and flutter kick creates irritation of the extensor tendons of the foot and ankle at the level of the extensor retinaculum, producing pain. Tinea pedis (athlete's foot) usually presents with itching rather than pain. Ankle sprains are not common in aquatic sports, and, when they occur, they are usually from slipping on a wet pool deck or in the locker room. Morton's neuroma is a painful interdigital neuroma of the common digital nerve between the metatarsals and is not associated with swimming. Tarsal navicular stress fractures are primarily seen in running and jumping sports.

79-4. e. Repetitive shoulder circumduction during swimming stretches the shoulder joint capsule, predisposing swimmers to shoulder instability. Although instability may be seen in swimmers with any of the strokes, backstroke swimmers are particularly susceptible to anterior instability ("apprehension shoulder") while doing backstroke turns with the arm abducted.

79-5. c. Otitis externa is inflammation of the external ear canal, which may present with ear swelling and discharge. It is caused by bacterial infection, fungal infection, or irritants such as pool chemicals or systemic allergies. It is commonly seen in aquatic sports due to retained moisture in the ear and is termed *swimmer's ear*. Cotton in the ears will absorb water while swimming, and this is not recommended. Wearing hard ear plugs or using cotton swabs in the ears can damage the ear canal epithelium and remove the protective cerumen, predisposing the athlete to infection. Silicone ear plugs provide superior protection. Antibiotic drops should be used cautiously and rarely as prophylaxis to decrease the risk of sensitivity to the medication. Prevention helps to decrease swimmer's ear. Placing a drying agent such as acetic acid in the ear after each pool session is a good drying method. Other methods include head tilting to extrude water or holding a blow dryer (on low setting) 7 inches from the ear.

CHAPTER **80**

Overhand Throwing Sports
Robert E. Sallis, MD

QUESTIONS

80-1. The correct sequence of the throwing motion is:
    a. acceleration, cocking, release and deceleration, follow-through.
    b. cocking, acceleration, release and deceleration, follow-through.
    c. cocking, follow-through, acceleration, release and deceleration.
    d. follow-through, cocking, acceleration, release and deceleration.
    e. acceleration, cocking, follow-through, release and deceleration.

80-2. The "dead arm syndrome":
    a. is characterized by a complete paralysis of the throwing arm.
    b. is the result of a torn rotator cuff.
    c. is often associated with a fracture of the midshaft of the humerus.
    d. is usually associated with an anterior labrum tear.
    e. is caused by inadequate flexibility.

80-3. Throwers with stage II impingement syndrome have all of the following, EXCEPT:
    a. a painful arc in their abduction motion between 80 and 120 degrees.
    b. true weakness of the rotator cuff.
    c. pain that is worse with overhead activity.
    d. symptoms of rotator cuff and/or biceps tendinitis.
    e. all of the above are correct.

80-4. With regards to shoulder instability in throwers, which is false?
    a. laxity refers to normal glenohumeral translation.
    b. instability is helpful in pitchers who throw with tremendous velocity.
    c. instability may be congenital.
    d. glenohumeral instability may lead to the impingement syndrome.
    e. b and c.

80-5. Regarding elbow injuries in throwers, which statement is correct?
    a. throwing causes a valgus stress at the elbow.
    b. the medial elbow is subject to compressive forces with throwing.
    c. the lateral elbow is subject to tensile stresses with throwing.
    d. maximal stress at the elbow is produced by the cocking phase of the throwing motion.
    e. all of the above.

ANSWERS

80-1. b. The correct sequence of the four phases of the throwing motion is cocking, acceleration, release and deceleration, follow-through.

80-2. d. The "dead arm syndrome" refers to a sudden paralyzing pain that occurs during the cocking phase of the throwing motion. This is usually the result of an anterior labrum tear, which allows subluxation of the humeral head and irritation of the brachial plexus.

80-3. b. True weakness of the rotator cuff is indicative of a cuff tear. This is the end stage (stage III) of the impingement syndrome, which produces all of the other symptoms listed.

80-4. b. Instability is abnormal translation (i.e., subluxation or dislocation) at the glenohumeral joint. This movement can irritate the rotator cuff tendons, leading to tendinitis and the impingement syndrome. Instability may be congenital, the result of traumatic dislocation, or repetitive overuse. Laxity is normal translation at the glenohumeral joint and may be increased in pitchers.

80-5. a. Throwing causes a valgus stress at the elbow that is maximal during the acceleration phase. This produces tensile stresses medially (at the ulnar collateral ligament) and compressive forces laterally (at the radiocapitellar joint).

CHAPTER **81**

Skiing Injuries

Steven D. Stahle, MD

Robert J. Dimeff, MD

QUESTIONS

81-1. A skier who presents with uncontrolled shivering and who appears pale and cool with a temperature of 34°C is probably suffering from:
a. acute mountain sickness.
b. severe hypothermia.
c. mild hypothermia.
d. frostnip.

81-2. Innovations in ski boots and bindings have decreased injuries in all of the following areas, EXCEPT:
a. ankle sprains.
b. tibial fractures.
c. anterior cruciate ligament (ACL) tears.
d. ankle fractures.

81-3. "Skier's thumb" is a common injury seen on the slopes. The most common mechanism of this injury is:
a. snowboarding and falling forward.
b. skiing for multiple hours on consecutive days.
c. fastening ski boots in preparation to ski.
d. falling down with a ski pole in the hand trying to break a fall.

81-4. Which type of injuries accounts for 75% of all reported cross-country injuries?
   a. overuse injuries.
   b. head and neck injuries.
   c. tibial fractures.
   d. ACL tears.

81-5. Which type of skiing is the world's fastest growing winter sport and has a high incidence of upper extremity injuries?
   a. alpine skiing.
   b. snowboarding.
   c. cross-country skiing.
   d. free-style skiing.

ANSWERS

81-1. c. Mild hypothermia presents as above with a core temperature of 32°-35°C. With moderate and severe hypothermia shivering usually stops as temperature decreases. Mental status changes can be seen along with vital sign changes. Acute mountain sickness presents differently and is not related to temperature, although they can both occur in the same type of climate. Frostnip is a localized itching, swelling, and sometimes painful erythema caused by mild frostbite.

81-2. c. Higher, stiffer boots plus release bindings have dramatically reduced ankle sprains and leg injuries, especially fractures. ACL injuries, however, have increased and continue to be problematic for the skier. ACL tears account for roughly two-thirds of knee injuries in skiers.

81-3. d. Ulnar collateral ligament (UCL) sprains of the first metacarpophalangeal joint are common in skiers who use poles. UCL sprains occur when valgus force is applied to the thumb, usually during a fall while holding on to a ski pole. This injury occurs less often in snowboarders because they do not use ski poles. The injury is not related to extensive training or preparation to ski.

81-4. a. Overuse injuries are the most common injury in cross-country skiers. Head and neck trauma is rare. Tibial fractures and ACL tears are uncommon in cross-country skiers.

81-5. b. Snowboarding has tremendous popularity, and most injuries occur in young, inexperienced male riders. The skier is positioned sideways on the board, increasing the potential for injury to the forward limb. Wrist fractures are also commonly diagnosed in snowboarders due to impact on the upper extremity related to falls. Low back strains are also common.

CHAPTER **82**

Dance

C. Mark Chassay, MD

QUESTIONS

82-1. Which of the following dance team members makes aware and counsels regarding the physical limitations of dancers in addition to providing references for proper technique?
a. artistic director.
b. instructor.
c. therapist.
d. physician.

82-2. The most common underlying characteristic for developing menstrual disorders such as amenorrhea is:
a. stress.
b. inadequate nutrition.
c. low body fat.
d. low estrogen levels.

82-3. The leg disorder characterized by deep pain in the gluteal region, which worsens on climbing stairs, moving from sitting to standing, increased activity, and even prolonged sitting, is:
a. greater trochanter bursitis.
b. piriformis syndrome.
c. tendinitis.
d. degenerative joint disease of the hip.

82-4. Which ankle impingement disorder is characterized by tenderness and swelling between the lateral malleolus and extensor digitorum communis? It is sometimes mistaken for "tight" heel-cords:
   a. anterior impingement.
   b. posterior impingement.

82-5. Dancer's fracture radiographically yields a:
   a. stress fracture.
   b. linear fracture.
   c. spiral fracture.

ANSWERS

82-1. b. Instructors also provide their pupils with direction in proper conditioning, strengthening, and nutrition. Artistic directors, on the other hand, plan tours and ensure ideal dance floor conditions and availability, in addition to assisting in matching dance requirements with each athlete's capabilities.

82-2. c. All are important in the multifactorial causes; however, the most common underlying characteristic is low body fat. At least 17% body fat is required for menarche, whereas 22% is generally required for resumption of menses after secondary amenorrhea.

82-3. b. Piriformis syndrome is essentially a diagnosis of exclusion; it is associated with overuse syndromes and related to weak and/or inadequate external rotation due to the entrapment of the sciatic nerve.

82-4. a. Anterior impingement by extreme dorsiflexion can also cause pain and weakness, but the most usual complaint by the athlete is lack of full depth on plié. The posterior impingement or dancer's heel is caused by extreme plantar flexion and exhibits posterior symptoms. Posterior impingement is sometimes mistaken for Achilles' tendinitis.

82-5. c. This spiral fracture of the fifth metatarsal shaft is best treated by short immobilization with gradual increase in activity and later protection from further injury. The mechanism of injury is by inversion on pointe in the dancer.

INDEX

A

Acclimation, altitude, 66-68
Achilles tendon, 232, 234, 286, 287
Acquired immunodeficiency syndrome, 21-25
Acromioclavicular arthrosis, 125
Acromioclavicular joint, 120, 122
Acute mountain sickness, 66, 68
Adolescent, 101-103
  growth in, 264-266
  musculoskeletal injuries in, 246-251
  rehabilitation for, 252-254
  strength training for, 254-257
AIDS, 21-25
Allergic reaction, of skin, 48
Amenorrhea, 82-84, 90, 91, 93
  dancer and, 298, 300
Amnesia, retrograde, 168
Amphetamine, 116, 117, 118
Anabolic steroid, 108, 112-115
Anabolism, 114
Androgenic steroid, 112-115
Anemia, 18-20
Ankle
  anatomy of, 218-220
  basketball injury of, 278, 280
  bracing of, 243-245, 274
  dancing and, 299, 300
  fracture of, 226-228
  ligament injury to, 221-225
  rehabilitation of, 229-231
  swimming and, 289, 290
  taping of, 243-245, 274
Anorexia nervosa, 91, 94
Anterior cruciate ligament injury, 194-201
  in child, 250
AO classification of ankle fracture, 228
Apprehension shoulder, 289, 290
Aquatic sports, 288-291
Arch, medial, 285, 287
Arrhythmia, 12-14
Arthritis, acromioclavicular, 125
Arthrosis, acromioclavicular, 125
Asthma, exercise-induced, 32-34
Athletic heart syndrome, 15
Auricular hematoma, 53
Avulsion
  hip, 215, 217
  tooth, 53
Avulsion fracture, in child, 252, 254

B

Back pain, 183-185; see also Spine
  pregnancy and, 87
  spondylolysis and, 186-190
BakerÕs cyst, 206, 208-209
Balke-Ware protocol, 11
Band, iliotibial, 269
Banned drug, 107-109
BAPS system, 229, 231
Barotrauma, 53
Basal body temperature, 62
Baseball injury, 127-128, 131
  in child, 238, 251
Basketball injury, 278-280
  back, 188, 190
Beta-adrenergic blocking agent, 111
Beta-2-agonist, asthma and, 34
Biceps brachii muscle, 144, 146
Biceps femoris muscle, 269
Bicycling injury, 281-284
Biomechanical ankle platform system board, 229, 231
Biomechanics of running, 235-239
Black heel, 49
Bleeding
  epistaxis and, 51-52
  gastrointestinal, 40
  stress hematuria and, 19, 20
Blood doping, 18-20
Blood supply to hip, 212, 214
Body fat, 300
Body temperature
  cold-related disorder and, 58-65
  heat-related disorder and, 54-57
Bone
  of child, 246, 249
  female athlete and, 93
  growth of, 264, 266
  osteoporosis and, 95-97
Boot, ski, 295, 297
Boutoni"re deformity, pseudo-, 161
Brachial plexus injury, 135-137

football and, 276
Brachioradialis reflex, 146
Bracing
  ankle, 243-245, 274, 276
  spinal, 189
Bruce protocol, 9
Bruise, 275, 276
Bucket handle tear of meniscus, 204
Buckle fracture, 249
Bulimia nervosa, 91, 94
Burner, 179, 181
Burnout, 76, 78
Butterfly stroke, 131

C

Calcaneal apophysitis, 232, 234
Calcaneus, 220
Calcium, amenorrhea and, 82
Canal, GuyonÕs, 157, 162-163, 284
Carbohydrate, 79
Cardiac arrhythmia, 12-14
Cardiac rehabilitation, 2-4
Cardiomyopathy, hypertrophic, 15
Carpal fracture, 154, 160
Carpal tunnel syndrome, 151, 152
Cerebellar testing, 168
Cerebral edema, 68
Cervical spine, 169-185; *see also* Spine, cervical
Child, 101-103, 246-257
  musculoskeletal injuries in, 246-251
  rehabilitation for, 252-254
  strength training for, 254-257
Chlamydia trachomatis, 27, 28
Chondral injury, 251
Chondromalacia patella, 204, 206, 208
Cocaine, 109, 116, 117, 118
Cold-related disorder, 58-65
Collateral ligament
  of knee, 195, 196
  ulnar, 143
    skierÕs thumb and, 161
    tear of, 151, 152
Compartment disorder, 241
Compression
  ankle injury and, 231
  ulnar nerve, 284
Concussion, 164-165
Conduction heat loss, 63
Consciousness
  in child, 246, 249
  in head injury, 164-165, 166, 168
Contraction, eccentric muscle, 236, 240
Convection heat loss, 63
Coracoacromial ligament, 130
Coracoclavicular ligament, 122
Coracoid process fracture, 133, 134
Coronary heart disease, 2-4, 71
Corticosteroid, banned, 110-111

Cross country, 296, 297
Cruciate ligament injury, 194-201
  in child, 250
Cycling injury to shoulder, 133, 134
Cyst, BakerÕs, 206, 208-209

D

Dance, 298-300
Danis-Weber classification of ankle fracture, 227, 228
Dead arm syndrome, 292, 294
Death, sudden, 15-17
Deltoid ligament, 220, 222, 224
Dermatological disorder, 48-50
Diabetes mellitus, 35-37
Diet, 79-81
Dilutional pseudoanemia, 20
Dimethyl sulfoxide, 105, 106
Disk surgery, 184, 185
Dislocation
  cervical spine, 173-175
  elbow, 148, 149
  glenohumeral, 139, 140
  patellar, 250
  shoulder, 132-134
Dissociation, scapholunate, 153-154, 158-159, 260
Diving accident, 169, 170, 172, 174, 175
  in child, 246, 249
Diving injury, 289, 290
Doping, blood, 18-20
Dorsal hood injury, 163
Down syndrome, 288, 290
Drop test, 126
Drug
  banned, 107-109
  illicit, 116-118
Drug therapy
  antiinflammatory, 104-106
  asthma and, 32-34
  hypertension and, 5-6, 8

E

Ear
  disorder of, 51-53
  diving and, 289, 290
Eating disorder, 91, 98-100
Eccentric muscle contraction, 236, 240
Edema, altitude-related, 68
Elbow injury, 141-149
  in child, 238, 251
  overuse, 262, 263
  throwing and, 293, 294
Elderly athlete, 45-47
  shoulder injury in, 124, 125
Electrocardiography, 12-14
Elevation for ankle injury, 231
Emptying, gastric, 39, 40

Endurance training, 73, 74
Energy, 79
Enhancement, performance, 77, 78
Environmental disorder
    altitude-related, 66-68
    cold-related, 58-65
    heat-related, 54-57
Epicondylitis, 142, 143, 145, 146, 147, 149
Epidemiology of injuries, 271-273
Epiphyseal fracture, 257, 260
Epistaxis, 53
Estrogen deficiency, 93
Evaporation, 63
Exercise physiology, 72-75
Exercise testing, 9-11
Exercise-associated amenorrhea, 82-84
Exercise-induced asthma, 32-34
Exercise-induced hematuria, 43, 44
Exhaustion, 72
Extensor carpi radialis brevis, 143
Extraaxial cervical spine injury, 176-178
Eye injury, 279, 280

F

FABERE test, 214
Fat, 81
    body, 300
Female athlete, 82-100
    eating disorder in, 91, 94, 98-100
    menstrual disorder and, 82-84
    osteoporosis in, 95-97
    pregnancy and, 85-89
    triad of disorders in, 90-94
Femoral neck fracture, 215, 217
Femoral physis, 264, 266
Ferritin, 20
Fibrocartilage complex, triangular, 160
Fibula stress fracture, 228
Fibular squeeze test, 221, 224
Field management
    of cervical spine injury, 179-182
    of fracture, 258-259, 260
    of head injury, 166-168
Fifth metatarsal injury, 151, 152
    in dancer, 300
Finger
    injury to, 142, 143
    jammed, 154, 161
    mallet, 151, 152, 162
    weakness of, 150, 152
Flexibility deficit, 267-270
Flexion
    of elbow, 141, 142, 143
    forearm, 144, 146
    plantar, 290
Flexion contracture of hip, 212, 214
Fluids, 80, 81
Foot
    anatomy of, 218-220
    injury to, 232-234

swimming and, 289, 290
Football injury, 274-276
    brachial plexus, 135, 137
    epidemiology of, 272
    head, 166, 168
    knee, 199, 200-201
    shoulder, 133, 134
    spinal, 169-172, 173, 175, 179-182
Force
    in biomechanics of running, 235, 240
    unconsciousness and, 168
Forearm and elbow, 141-149
Fracture
    ankle, 226-228
    carpal, 154, 160
    cervical spine, 173-175
    coracoid process, 133, 134
    dancerÕs, 299
    epiphyseal, 257
    femoral neck, 215, 217
    hamate, 160
    hip, 215, 217
    management of, 258-263
    metacarpal, 155, 161, 162
    pars articularis, 189
    phalangeal, 161
    radial head, 148, 149
    scaphoid, 150-151, 152, 158, 160, 163,
        280
    stress, 241
    tibial, 250
    wrist, 258, 260
Frostbite, 60-61

G

Gait, biomechanics of, 235-239
Gait cycle, 218, 220
GamekeeperÕs thumb, 152
Gastric emptying, 39, 40
Gastrointestinal disorder, 38-41
Genitourinary disorder, 42-44
Geriatric athlete, 45-47
Glenohumeral dislocation, 139, 140
Glenohumeral ligament, 122
Glucose, 35-37
Glycogen, 74, 81
Growth, 264-266
Growth hormone, 111
GuyonÕs canal, 157, 162-163, 284
Gymnastics
    back pain in, 187, 189
    hyperextension of knee and, 247,
        250
    wrist injury to, 154, 159
Gynecomastia, 114-115

H

Hamate fracture, 160

Hamstring stretching, 272, 273
Hand
  cycling injury to, 282
  examination of, 150-152
  injury to, 153-163
Head
  humeral, 132, 134
  nodding of, 176, 178
  radial, 148, 149, 259, 260
Head injury
  concussion and, 164-165
  field management of, 166-168
  mild, 274, 276
Heart disease, 2-4
Heart rate, 72, 74
Heat disorder, 54-57
Heel, black, 49
Heel pain, 232-233, 234
Helmet, football, 179, 180, 181
Hematology, 18-20
Hematoma, 275, 276
  auricular, 53
Hematuria, 44
  exercise-induced, 43, 44
  stress, 19, 20
Herpes, in wrestler, 48
Herpes gladiatorum, 30, 31, 49
Hip
  anatomy of, 212, 214
  examination of, 212-214
  injury to, 215-217
Hockey, back pain and, 187, 189
Hood, dorsal, 163
Hook of hamate fracture, 160
Hormone, amenorrhea and, 83
Human immunodeficiency virus infection,
  21-25
Humeral head dislocation, 132, 134
Humerus, 120, 122
Hydration, 80
Hypercholesterolemia, 16
Hyperextension, of knee, 194, 196, 247,
  250
Hyperflexion of cervical spine, 169-170, 172
Hyperlordosis, 189
Hypertension, 5-7
Hyperthermia, pregnancy and, 86
Hypertrophic cardiomyopathy, 15
Hyperventilation, altitude and, 68
Hypoestrogenemia, 91
Hypothermia, 58-65, 297

I

Ice, for ankle injury, 231
Iliotibial band, 269
Illicit drug, 116-118
Imaging
  ankle, 222, 224
  back pain and, 189, 190
  of head injury, 165
  of knee, 208
  knee injury and, 200

Immunodeficiency, 21-25
Impetigo, 48
Impingement
  ankle, 278, 280
    dancing and, 299, 300
  shoulder, 125, 127-129
    in child, 248
    throwing sports and, 292, 294
Infection, 29-31
  HIV, 21-25
  sexually transmitted, 26-28
Inflammation of ear, 290-291
Injury
  baseball, 127-128, 131
  basketball, 278-280
  bicycling, 281-284
  cycling, 133, 134
  epidemiology of, 271-273; *see also specific*
    type of injury
  football, 274-276
  rotator cuff, 125, 127-131
  skiing, 295-297
  volleyball, 128, 131
Instability, shoulder, 132-134
  in child, 250-251
  throwing and, 293, 294
Interphalangeal joint, proximal, 156, 162-
  163
Intersection syndrome, 151, 152, 154, 159
Iron deficiency anemia, 18

J

Jammed finger, 154, 161
Joint
  acromioclavicular, 120, 122
  proximal interphalangeal, 156, 162-163
  radioulnar, 143
  sacroiliac, 213, 214
JumperÕs knee, 207, 209

K

Knee injury, 194-211
  anterior knee pain and, 205-209
  cycling injury to, 281-282, 283
  hyperextension, in child, 247, 250
  ligamentous, 197-201
  mechanism of, 194-196
  meniscal, 195, 196, 202-204
  rehabilitation of, 210-211
  running and, 286, 287
  swimming and, 288, 290

L

LachmanÕs test, 198, 200
Laryngeal trauma, 52
Lateral collateral ligament of knee, 195,
  196

Lateral epicondylitis, 142, 143, 145, 146, 147, 149
Legg-Perthes disease, 247, 250
Ligament
  ankle, 221-225
  anterior cruciate, in child, 250
  coracoacromial, 130
  coracoclavicular, 122
  cruciate, 194-201
  deltoid, 220, 222, 224
  elbow, 145, 146
  glenohumeral, 122
  lateral collateral, 195, 196
  ulnar collateral, 143
    skierÕs thumb and, 161
    tear of, 151, 152
Limb length discrepancy, 212, 214
Log-rolling, 180, 181
Low back pain, 183-185
  spondylolysis and, 186-190
Lower extremity; *see also* Ankle; Foot; Knee
  shin splints and, 236-239, 241-242
Lumbar spine, 183-193; *see also* Spine, lumbar

M

Malalignment, in knee, 208, 209
Mallet finger, 151, 152, 162
Marijuana, 118
Maxillofacial trauma, 53
Medial arch pain, 285, 287
Median nerve, 143
Menarche, 91, 93
Meniscal injury, 195, 196, 202-204
  in child, 250
Menopause, 97
Menstrual disorder, 82-84
  in dancer, 298, 300
Meralgia paraesthetica, 216, 217
Metacarpal fracture, 155, 161, 162
Metacarpophalangeal joint, 161-162
Metatarsal fracture, 300
Mitral valve prolapse, 10, 11
Muscle
  contraction of, 236, 240
  football injury to, 275, 276
Musculoskeletal growth, 264-266
Myositis ossificans, 216, 217
  of elbow, 147, 149

N

Nasal disorder, 51-53
Navicular, 219, 220
Neck, femoral, 215, 217
Neck injury, 169-172, 174, 175
  cycling, 282, 284
Neisseria gonorrhoeae, 26, 28
Nerve
  cervical, 178
  median, 143
  radial, 162-163
  ulnar, cycling and, 284
Nerve root, 144, 146, 181
Nodding of head, 176, 178
Nodule, Achilles, 287
Nonsteroidal antiinflammatory drug, 104-106
Numbness of finger, 150, 152
Nutrition, 79-81

O

Older athlete, 45-47
Orthotic, for runner, 236, 240
Osgood-Schlatter disease, 250
Osteochondritis dissecans
  in child, 246, 249
  of elbow, 147, 149
Osteoporosis, 95-97
Otitis externa, 290-291
Ottawa ankle rules, 221, 224
Overhand throwing, 121, 122, 292-294
Overuse injury, 261-263
  in child, 246, 249
  cycling and, 283-284
  to knee, 205-211
  skiing and, 297

P

Pain
  ankle, 223, 224
  flexibility and, 268
  heel, 232-233, 234
  hip, 214
  knee, 205-211; *see also* Knee injury
  low back, 183-185
  lumbar spine, 191-193
  running and, 285-287
  spondylolysis and, 186-190
Paresthesia, 282
Pars interarticular, 183, 184, 185
Patellar injury, 195, 196
  in child, 250
  epidemiology of, 272
Patellofemoral stress syndrome, 286, 287
Patrick test, 214
Pectoralis major muscle, 122
Pediatric athlete, 101-103, 246-257
  musculoskeletal injuries in, 246-251
  rehabilitation for, 252-254
  strength training for, 254-257
Performance enhancement, 77, 78
Periostitis, 241-242
Phalangeal fracture, 161
PhalenÕs test, 156-163, 163
Physiology, exercise, 72-75
Physis, femoral, 264, 266
Piriformis syndrome, 216, 217
Pisiform fracture, 160
Plantar flexion, 290

Plexus, brachial, 135-137
Polycythemia, 68
Popliteus tendon, 208
Postconcussion syndrome, 167, 168
Posterior cruciate ligament, 196
Posterior tibial muscle, 232, 234
Posterior tibial tendon, 234
Pregnancy, 85-89
Premature ventricular contraction, 13
Preparticipation examination, 69-71
Prepubescent athlete, 101-103, 257; *see
    also* Child
Prescription, exercise, 9-11
Prolapse, mitral valve, 10, 11
Pronation, elbow, 141, 143
Prophylactic bracing of ankle, 274, 276
Protein, 79, 81
Proximal interphalangeal joint, 156, 162-
    163,
Pseudo-boutoni"ere deformity, 161
Psychology, sports, 76-78
Pulmonary disorder, 32-34
Pulmonary edema, 68

Q

Quadriceps
    of child, 254
    flexibility of, 268

R

Radial head fracture, 148, 149
Radial nerve, 162-163
Radiculopathy, 276
Radioulnar joint, 143
Radius fracture, 259, 260
    in child, 249
Rectus femoris muscle, 269
Reflex, brachioradialis, 146
Rehabilitation
    ankle, 229-231
    cardiac, 2-4
    for child, 252-254
    knee, 210-211
    lumbar spine pain and, 191-193
    overuse injury and, 261, 263
    shoulder, 138-140
Renal disorder, 42-44
Respiration, heat loss and, 63
Rest
    ankle injury and, 231
    stiffness and, 270
Retrograde amnesia, 168
Return to play
    after head injury, 164-168
    lumbar spine pain and, 191-193
rhEPO, 20
RICE, 231
Root, nerve, 181

Rotation
    ankle, 228
    cervical, 176, 178
    shoulder, 120, 121, 122
Rotator cuff injury, 125, 127-129
    throwing and, 294
Running
    biomechanics of, 235-239
    injury from, 285-287
Rupture of central slip of extensor tendon,
    161

S

Sacroiliac joint, 213, 214
Saddle, bicycle, 281, 283
Scaphoid fracture, 150-151, 152, 158, 160,
    163, 280
Scapholunate dissociation, 153-154, 158-
    159, 260
Scapular, 121, 122
Second impact syndrome, 166, 168
Semimembranosus bursa, 208-209
Semimembranosus tendinitis, 278, 280
Sexually transmitted disease, 26-28
Shin splints, 236-239, 241-242
Shoulder, 120-140
    anatomy and biomechanics of, 120-122
    brachial plexus injury and, 135-137
    in child, 248, 250-251
    examination of, 123-126
    football injury to, 275, 276
    impingement of
        rotator cuff injury and, 125, 127-129
        throwing sports and, 292, 294
    instability of, 132-134
        in child, 250-251
        throwing and, 293, 294
    rehabilitation of, 138-140
    rotator cuff injury to, 125, 127-131
    swimming and, 289, 290
Sickle cell trait, 19, 20
Sit and reach test, 269
Skateboard injury, 226, 228
SkierÕs thumb, 152, 155, 161, 295, 297
Skiing injury, 295-297
Skin disorder, 48-50
Snowboarding, 297
Soccer injury, 226-227, 228
Spine
    cervical, 169-185
        anatomy and biomechanics of, 169-
            172
        in child, 246, 249
        extraaxial injury to, 176-178
        field management of, 179-182
        fracture and dislocation of, 173-175
    lumbar, 183-193
        low back pain and, 183-185
        rehabilitation of, 191-193

spondylolysis and spondylolisthesis and, 185-190
Splinting of fracture, 260
Splints, shin, 236, 241
Spondylolisthesis, 184, 185, 186-190, 247, 250
Spondylolysis, 186-190
Sports psychology, 76-78
Sprain
  ankle, 222, 224
  lumbar spine, 192, 193
Squeeze test, fibular, 221, 224
Stacking, 114
Standing toe touch test, 269
Steroid, anabolic, 108, 112-115
Stinger, 179, 181
Strength training, for child, 255-257
Stress, tibial, 237-238, 241
Stress fracture, 241, 262, 263
  fibular, 228
Stress hematuria, 19, 20
Stretching
  for child, 253, 254
  flexibility and, 268, 272, 273
Sudden death, 15-17
Supination, elbow, 141, 143
Supraspinatus tendinitis, 131
Surgery, ankle, 226, 228
Swelling, of knee, 248, 250
Swimming, 288-291
  shoulder injury and, 129, 131
Syphilis, 26

T

T₃, 100
Taping, ankle, 243-245
Tear
  anterior cruciate ligament, 198, 200
  meniscal, 202-204
  rotator cuff, 125
Temperature-related disorder
  cold, 58-65
  heat, 54-57
Tendinitis
  patellar, 272
  semimembranosus, 278, 280
  supraspinatus, 131
Tendon
  Achilles, 286, 287
  popliteus, 208
  posterior tibial, 234
Tennis
  elbow injury in, 142, 143
  shoulder injury in, 124, 125
Teres major muscle, 122
Testicular torsion, 44
Testosterone, 108, 110
Threshold, ventilatory, 73, 75
Throat disorder, 51-53
Throwing, 292-294

overuse injury from, 261, 263
  shoulder injury and, 129, 131
Thumb, skierÕs, 152, 155, 161, 295, 297
Thyroxine, eating disorder and, 100
Tibial muscle, posterior, 232, 234
Tibial stress injury, 237-238, 241, 261, 263
Tibial tendon, posterior, 234
Tibialis anterior muscle, 218, 220
Tilt board system, 229, 231
TinelÕs sign, 163
Tooth avulsion, 53
Torsion, testicular, 44
Torus fracture, 249
Track injury, ankle, 227, 228
Training
  endurance, 73, 74
  strength, for child, 255-257
  weight
    for child, 253, 254, 256, 257
    for elderly, 46, 47
Traumatic urethritis, 43, 44
Treponema pallidum, 26, 28
Triad of disorders in female athlete, 90-94
Triangular fibrocartilage complex, 160
Triplane ankle fracture, 228

U

Ulnar collateral ligament, 143
  skierÕs thumb and, 161
  tear of, 151, 152
Ulnar nerve injury, 282, 284
Unconsciousness, 164-165, 166, 168
  in child, 246, 249
Urethritis, traumatic, 43, 44
Urine testing, 108

V

Valgus angle, 146
Valgus instability of elbow, 141, 143
Vascular system of hip, 212, 214
Ventilation, altitude and, 68
Ventilatory threshold, 73, 75
Vitamin, 80, 81
Volleyball, shoulder injury and, 123-124, 125
Volleyball injury, shoulder, 128, 131

W

Walking, 235-236, 240
Weight lifting, 123, 125
Weight training
  for child, 253, 254, 256, 257
  in elderly, 46, 47
Wrestler, herpes in, 48
Wrist
  examination of, 150-152